herpes:

WHAT TO DO WHEN YOU HAVE IT

by Oscar Gillespie, PhD

Cofounder of New York Help

A GD/PERIGEE BOOK

Perigee Books
are published by
The Putnam Publishing Group
200 Madison Avenue
New York, New York 10016

Library of Congress catalog card number: 81-85484
ISBN 0-399-50827-9

First Perigee printing, 1983
One previous Grosset & Dunlap printing
Printed in the United States of America
1 2 3 4 5 6 7 8 9

Design by John M-Röblin

Contents

Contents

Introduction

Herpes is a disease currently shrouded in more myths, misinformation, and emotional connotations than perhaps any other health problem. A disease that cannot be cured outright and that can reappear at some time in the future after it has been contracted is reason enough for genuine concern, even when its symptoms are for the most part not physically serious. But since these symptoms most often are on the genitals, it is not just our body that is threatened but also our sexuality—our feelings about ourselves and about being physically close to another human being.

Until recently, due to the lack of information as well as the fact that herpes cannot be cured, many people who contracted the virus either ignored it or hid the fact. Ignoring herpes undoubtedly contributed to its spread in the population. And individuals choosing to hide it had to carry a secret burden around with them, which, as you can imagine, had quite an impact on their interpersonal lives. A few others were lucky enough to get sufficient information to be able to solve whatever difficulties herpes presented to them.

HERPES: WHAT TO DO WHEN YOU HAVE IT clarifies the issues surrounding herpes—its treatments and emotional implications. The information herein will provide the means for you to deal effectively with herpes should you have it, contract it in the future, or become involved in some way with someone who has it. Its aim is to help you avoid, or at least drastically reduce, your experience of the pitfalls and syndromes that have become associated with herpes for one reason or another, so that you can live your life and enjoy your relationships with as much freedom as possible.

Today, people are less willing to hide their frustrations about potential interruptions in their personal and sexual lives and are more prepared to ask questions about events that affect their well-being. This healthy rebellion is not confined to herpes, but it has played a large role in bringing herpes to the attention of both physicians and public.

The change in attitude is due partly to the more candid exploration of sexuality in the last two decades and partly to a reevaluation of what is important for a free, full, and healthy life. Being healthy doesn't mean just the absence of disease symptoms but also includes feeling good emotionally and socially. Good interpersonal relationships are one of the most important determinants of well-being, and as such require just as much attention as is paid to physical symptoms. An illness that, for whatever reason, disrupts the capacity to be intimate with another human being is very serious indeed. So herpes is beginning to be recognized as a disease in the *quality* of life—quite a step forward.

The more honest appraisal of sexuality has had other effects as well. An important one is that a small dent has been made in the stigmas associated with sexual difficulties and sexual diseases. The dent has made it easier for people to seek help when something is not right. However, the taboo associated with sexual diseases has not ended yet, and since there is no cure for herpes, it has acquired its own stigma as "the one to avoid at all costs" or "the worst of them all." This is generated, again, by lack of knowledge and understanding.

The media has played a leading role here, bringing a mixed blessing to the herpes problem as it exists today. The media has helped considerably to alert physicians, researchers, and the general public to the dimensions of the problem—a very fine public service. But the issue has been dramatically overplayed with a sensationalism sufficient to instill a profound fear in anyone who contracts herpes or becomes involved with someone who already has it. Articles featuring selected information and used for maximum impact have been responsible for as much irrationality about herpes as the lack of information and understanding was in the past. A small percentage of men and women indeed do run into serious difficulties after contracting herpes, until they get on top of the disease. These difficulties are prolonged in far too many cases for want of a realistic and therapeutic presentation of information.

Many people can read the scientific literature, some can interpret it, and a few can present it in human terms to others in a therapeutic way. HERPES: WHAT TO DO WHEN YOU HAVE IT reflects both the scientific facts as well as the experiences of the men and women who came to me or NY HELP for clarification and aid after contracting herpes.

NY HELP is a local chapter of a national program initiated by the American Social Health Association (ASHA), a private organization dedicated to the control of sexually transmissible diseases. Recognizing the need for information and counseling about herpes, ASHA founded the

Herpes Resource Center, with a main goal of bringing medical and research attention to the herpes problem. This has been largely successful. Another goal was to mobilize and facilitate local community involvement in the human aspects of herpes.

Along with several talented and dedicated groundbreakers, I headed up the New York assault on the generally vague and unenlightened state of affairs surrounding herpes. We set up a self-help framework to provide information, support when necessary, and a forum for sharing concerns and frustrations. Discussion groups were organized to help solve emotional or interpersonal problems that herpes sufferers had run into because of the climate of confusion and misinformation. We saw how people really can, with a little help, come through and out of the difficulties they encounter. This process is occurring in many parts of the country and shows quite clearly that while herpes may seem insurmountable at first, it is far from that. It is just another problem to be solved and for the vast majority a not too difficult one. I have seen several hundred men and women do it. If reading this book makes it still easier for you, then it will have done its job. It should.

1
Herpes Virus

Herpes is not a new problem. It is rarely life-threatening in a physical sense, nor terribly life-disturbing in most any other respect for individuals who contract it. For these reasons, as well as the fact that it is a sexually transmissible disease, herpes has been essentially hidden from public attention until quite recently. However, access to correct information about herpes is the key to prevention and to the elimination of feelings of confusion and fear.

What is Herpes I and II?

Herpes is a viral infection that causes a rash on the skin or mucous membranes of the body. The most common form of herpes, occurring at some point in the lives of nearly ninety percent of the United States population, is the "cold sore" or "fever blister" on the lip or side of the mouth. Less common, although still very prevalent, are infections on or around the genitals. Herpes of the face is caused by the herpes simplex virus type I (HSV I); herpes of the genitals by herpes simplex type II (HSV II). Strictly speaking, the type I version of the virus can show up on the genitals and type II on the face, or, for that matter, either of them can infect any part of the body. While the specific virus types causing facial or genital herpes can be distinguished biologically, for all intents and purposes the effect on your body is the same. Only the location is different.

TRANSMISSION Herpes I or II is originally contracted by direct physical contact with an infected sore on another person. Facial or lip herpes is most often transmitted by kissing someone with a cold sore. Children often contract herpes infections on the mouth, face or eyes from a well-meant, well-placed, but highly virulent kiss from someone with an active cold sore. Genital herpes is most often contracted during sexual intercourse with a person who has an active genital infection. For this reason, herpes is called a venereal disease, or, more correctly, a sexually transmitted disease.

The important things to remember are that transmission can occur only when the virus comes in direct contact with mucous membranes or with abrasions in the skin, and that the part of the body contacting the virus is the part that will become infected. In other words, the infection will be very localized. Some people develop "whitlow," or herpes on the finger, contracted by touching herpetic sores with their hand. Wrestlers and rugby players sometimes acquire infections on the neck, arms, or other areas, called appropriately enough "herpes gladiatorum."

Because the virus is transmitted by direct physical contact, it is possible to transfer the virus to another part of the body by self-inoculation—touching an active sore and passing on the virus. While this is not very common, the fingers and eyes are particularly vulnerable to self-transfer especially during a "primary" (first-time) infection, as opposed to a "recurrence," which is, as it sounds, a reactivation of the original infection.

One never "just develops" herpes. Although an infection may seem to have appeared out of the blue, it was transmitted either from another person or by self-transfer.

Sometimes people who contract herpes are puzzled as to how it could have happened: A genital infection shows up apparently from nowhere, with neither sexual partner aware of a history of herpes or of intimate contact with someone with herpes. As you can imagine, this situation can cause a good deal of frustration and difficulty between the partners.

There are two explanations for what happened. The first deals with the transmittal of the virus. Genital infections can often be traced back to a cold sore virus in one partner A , who transmitted the virus during oral sex or by fondling partner B, after touching the sore with a hand. Partner B can then pass the virus back to Partner A during intercourse. According to the figures available from studies of HSV I infections, somewhere between 10 to 16 percent of genital infections are most likely contracted in this way.

The second explanation deals with the relative severity of infection in a person carrying herpes. After contact with herpes sores, a person may not show enough, or may not be sufficiently disturbed by, evident body symptoms to realize he or she has contracted an infection. This is called a subclinical infection. No obvious symptoms may show for a long time—and possibly will never surface—but the virus is in fact in the person's body. However, under particular circumstances, which shall be examined in more detail in chapters 4, 8, and 9, a surface rash may appear, apparently from some mysterious source. Transmission to a partner then can occur. The appearance of the rash in this way is technically called a recurrence, since the primary infection actually occurred some time previously. Why this might occur will be clear from the next section on the symptoms and course of herpes infections.

> Points to Remember
> ○ Herpes is a viral infection that causes a rash on the body.
> ○ Herpes is highly contagious when on the surface of the body and is spread by direct physical contact, whether sexual or otherwise.
> ○ The two viruses causing herpes (herpes simplex virus type I and herpes simplex virus type II) cannot be picked up just by proximity to someone who has an infection. The viruses gain access to the body through mucous membranes or through abrasions in the skin.

Symptoms and Course of Herpes Infections

A genital herpes infection generally will show from two to twenty days after contact has taken place. The rash that occurs is fairly easily identified by a trained physician. Avoid self-diagnosis! Consulting a friend isn't a good idea (unless your friend urges you to seek proper diagnosis). You may be convinced you have herpes when in fact you have something else. There are other important reasons why self-diagnosis is not a good idea, which we will discuss in chapter 5.

The infection shows as a rash of red patches with white blister-like sores, usually in clusters. Genital herpes will usually make an appearance on or around the penis in men and the vagina in women. Internal lesions from primary infections can also occur in the mouth, vagina, cervix, or anus, or anywhere on the body where the virus first entered.

The rash is often accompanied by one or all of the following: pain and discomfort in the area of the infection, fever, headache. Pain or burning when urinating is common with genital herpes, as are swollen glands in the groin. Women may notice a mild vaginal discharge.

The severity of the individual symptoms, or episode, depends on several factors, which include the virus load (how much virus one is inoculated with), one's constitution, and one's general physical health when the infection begins. The range of distress is very broad, from a subclinical infection that is probably very common, where nothing or very little may be noticed, on up to a severe and prolonged illness. Indeed, some cases may be so severe that the rash covers the entire genital area, and the patient is ill enough and uncomfortable enough to require hospitalization. Fortunately, such an episode is a reaction only to a primary infection. The time from initial appearance of the rash until the area heals over with new cells is, in most cases, only two to three weeks. It should be emphasized that the symptoms from a primary infection will invariably be far more severe than those of any future episode.

Viruses need the resources of body cells to survive and reproduce. When the herpes virus first enters the body, it reproduces pretty freely in the surface cells. It can spread itself out across neighboring areas with the help of moisture and friction (which is why, as you will see, a herpes sufferer is told to keep the area dry and *not to rub*).

Unless you have already been exposed to a particular virus, your body is essentially defenseless for a time in preventing it from having a field day if it enters your body. It takes time for your body to mount defenses in the form of antibodies to attack and kill the virus and the cells invaded by it. If you are reasonably healthy, this process will occur quite efficiently. But if you are run down and your body resources somewhat depleted, the job will be more difficult. Once formed, specific antibodies will be present in the system from this time on. But first time around, the virus has free play for a while.

If you have been exposed to herpes, *see your physician as soon as you notice symptoms!* External symptoms are a definite warning. But also pay attention to other signs, such as a vaginal discharge, or pain or burning in the genital area or when urinating. Do not wait until symptoms disappear—because they will! The herpes virus will not.

Initial diagnosis is made on the basis of visual examination. Unless something is visible, there is not much for a physician to go on. A definitive verification of the presence of herpes is done by means of a viral culture test. If you and your physician are unsure about symptoms, do suggest a culture test.

A blood test like those for syphilis and gonorrhea will not help because until specific antibodies develop, nothing will show up to indicate herpes. And, if antibodies do show up in a blood test, this only indicates that you have been exposed to herpes at some time in the past, and not that you have an active infection now.

The reason to seek attention early when you notice symptoms is that current treatments, if applied early enough, can be quite effective in preventing viral replication and spread. If the activity of the virus is minimized as much as possible at this point, you can protect yourself from any kind of complication. When attacked by body defenses, the virus can escape into nerve cells, where it is safe, and can go into what is called a "latent" or "dormant" phase. Early treatment strives to eliminate as much virus as possible before that happens.

> Points to Remember:
> ○ A primary herpes infection can result in a number of effects ranging from subclinical states to severe and prolonged symptoms, depending on such factors as amount of virus transmitted, your constitution, and your general physical health.
> ○ In most cases, the first outbreak will be the worst experience you have with herpes and will pass with appropriate precautions and care.
> ○ Don't self-diagnose, or self-medicate. Get early attention.

Latency and Recurrences

Herpes is such a difficult disease to cure outright because although symptoms may be gone and the area of the rash healed, the virus still remains in the body in such a state that it may be reactivated to cause another rash on the surface of the body. After healing has occurred, the virus enters nerve endings near the initial rash, migrating away from the surface of the skin, and escaping the body defenses that can only operate in other tissue. The virus moves along the nerve cells to what is called the sacral ganglion (ganglion being a collection of nerve cell bodies) just outside the spinal cord, where it can coexist with the cells without any overt difficulties occurring. It settles down, quite content to avoid being annihilated. The best way to characterize the virus at this time is as dormant. In facial herpes, the same process occurs in the nerve cells that make up the trigeminal nerve of the face, leading the virus to its ganglion outside the base of the brain.

The dormant herpes virus can remain in this state indefinitely without causing damage and without causing infectious lesions on the surface of the body. In effect, you are cured of the impact of herpes in your life in general, including the problem of transmission, while you and the virus coexist more or less harmoniously. The herpes virus is like the virus causing warts, which also remains in your body after the warts have disappeared. There is, therefore, no cause for alarm at this point.

For many people, the latent state is essentially permanent, and no further symptoms will develop unless the balance between virus and body is dramatically disturbed. For others, however, the relationship does not remain so stable, and periodically the virus retraces its original escape route toward the body surface. If sufficient virus safely leaves the nerve cells to invade other tissue, a new rash will develop pretty much where the first one occurred. This is the beginning of a recurrent outbreak.

Recurrences are very different from primary infections in that the body now has a reservoir of antibodies to mobilize against the virus when it leaves its natural retreat. Generally speaking, recurrences are much less severe than first-time infections and should get increasingly less severe with each new episode.

Patterns of recurrence depend on many factors and vary with each person. Some figures suggest an average recurrence rate of three to five outbreaks a year, each of which lasts between four and ten days. But again, this can vary with each individual. Some people will rarely break out while others will break out quite regularly. The pattern may vary considerably even within individuals, with perhaps a series of breakouts in quick succession, followed by a period of months or years without any outbreak at all.

In general, if nothing hinders the body's adjustment to the virus, outbreak frequency and duration will continue to decrease, and few symptoms will show after a few years.

The ideal situation can be difficult to bring about, since there are many factors that contribute to recurrent outbreaks and their healing. Your job is to play as big a role as possible in keeping the virus as dormant as possible. You can facilitate the body's adaptation process to a large degree, although it does take some time. The chapters on recurrences and personal problems will address specifically how you can do this. And the first thing to remember is that correct information—supplied herein—will reduce the uncertainties, fears, and anxieties that may hinder this adaptation process. Then you will be on the road to a fast adjustment and control over the problem.

Points to Remember:
○ After an initial infection, the herpes virus retreats from body defenses into nerve cells and away from the body surface to remain in a latent state.
○ Various disturbances can reactivate the virus so that it migrates back to the original site of infection and causes a recurrent outbreak.
○ The recurrences will gradually become less severe, especially once you identify the factors that hinder and that facilitate your body's adaptation.

2
Getting Rid of the Pain

The pain and discomfort of herpes is always worst in the period of adjustment shortly after the contraction of a primary infection and, if you develop the recurrent form, during the first few recurrent outbreaks. This chapter is aimed at helping you through any discomforts you may have now while at the same time providing you with easy-to-apply comfort measures that you can develop into a set of habits for the future. While you want relief immediately, also keep in mind that you are working on an adjustment process so that herpes will become less and less disrupting or uncomfortable in the future.

For most people, the discomfort of herpes is more an annoying or disturbing set of sensations than sharp and acute pain, although it can be severe enough to keep some people home, interfering with work and social life.

Conquering herpes is a question of adjustment between you and the virus over time. It should not have to be a long time, unless there is a specific physical complication or immunological deficiency, neither of which is a factor in the vast majority of herpes infections. I have dealt with literally hundreds of people who have spent the better part of two years or more wrestling with the adjustment process when for almost everyone it can be accomplished in several months with the right information, therapeutic counseling, and proper action on the person's part.

The secret is to take good care of yourself, both physically and mentally, and to do everything possible to go on living your life as fully as ever—and that's really no secret. Alleviating the physical discomfort is the first step.

The discomfort can occur for several reasons. Everyone's experience is not the same. You will learn to identify your particular needs and what can be done about them.

The activity of the virus in the nerve cells before and during an outbreak will often cause dull uncomfortable aches in the general area. For example, some genital herpes sufferers have what feels like a strained muscle in one leg that is hard to locate specifically or tenderness in part or all of the groin.

Disruptions in surface cells as they are invaded and killed by virus and/or body defenses will cause tenderness and sensitivity in that tissue. General inflammation and hotness, sometimes described as a feeling of having the flu in part of the pelvic area, can also occur.

In some women, because of the location of the rash stinging or burning will occur when urine runs over it. Stinging, burning or sensitivity when urinating or defecating may also be experienced by both men and women from generalized inflammation and tenderness.

Since there is an active fight taking place between your body and the virus, there may be the general body malaise which accompanies other infections.

The last thing to understand is also that anxiety and worry can increase the experience of physical pain and discomfort directly!

Soothing the Pain

If the pain is severe, your physician may prescribe a short-term course of analgesics. This is usually only necessary in primary cases. In normal cases, prescription painkillers such as codeine or Demerol are not a good idea, since they often cause side effects (constipation or urinary retention), which in turn will increase the discomfort. Nausea and sedation may also occur. Except in extremely severe cases, you are working against yourself by using strong narcotic analgesics. If necessary, two aspirins every three hours will be helpful. Use Tylenol if you cannot tolerate aspirin. But don't be foolish. Consult your physician before trying anything.

Here are some easy ways to soothe the discomfort of genital herpes. Use what is most effective and easy to apply for you:

- Hold hot compresses on the rash area for a few minutes several times a day. Please, not so hot that you damage your skin.
- Using an ice pack also will be soothing and cooling for most people.
- Soothe by bathing, either in plain body temperature water or with Burows or Epsom salts added, which also will help dry the rash and keep the area clean. Do not overdo bathing to the point of causing skin disruptions, which may help the virus spread. Instead, take a short, soothing bath and then

gently dry the area. By all means go swimming. You'll not infect somebody by swimming in a pool. Just remove your wet bathing suit when you are finished and make sure you dry the infected area well. Some people find that using a hair dryer helps—not too hot and not too close.

o Dab with plain alcohol if the rash is external. This will relieve itching and help keep the area clean and dry. Remember, the virus dies when it dries. Topical Xylocaine available from your druggist will provide temporary cooling and soothing.

o Douche gently with plain tap water if lesions are inside the vagina. Do not use an astringent substance like vinegar or other commercial preparations.

o Cover the rash briefly while urinating, if it is located so that urine running over it causes discomfort. Drink lots of fluids to dilute urine acidity.

o Use tampons or minipads if there is a discharge from the cervix. Remember to change them frequently. Tampons can be safely worn during menstruation as usual.

o Wear loose clothes. Friction will aggravate the discomfort of genital herpes and retard healing of the rash. Tight designer jeans just might not be worth it. Women will find wearing long skirts instead of pants a great relief if chafing is a problem. Wear cotton underwear; nylon will work against you. This will probably not be necessary in the future when herpes is under control, but do everything to make yourself comfortable now. After cleaning and drying external rashes, a light dusting with talcum powder (preferably unscented) will help the chafing problem a great deal. Friction from vigorous sex or masturbation will also contribute to discomfort and retard healing. Be careful until the area is completely healed. It is very counterproductive to start the process all over again by abrading skin in the rash area.

Please—rest and relax. At the very least, slow down a little! Do not be so busy that you can't possibly spend a minute on yourself. That is part of what stress is all about— making sure your schedule always keeps you too busy to have any fun or relaxation in your day. There are *always* underlying reasons why people are too busy for themselves. Even a brief look at those reasons will go a long way towards improving *any* of the discomforts or disturbances of having herpes. When you find yourself continually feeling that you have too much to do or to worry about, take a look at your priorities. To help you in this there is a chart in Chapter 9.

The last important step is often a difficult one, but it doesn't have to be. Develop a fixed and consistent routine for your comfort measures with definite prescribed times for their application. Then **forget about herpes!** Don't let herpes control you, even for the short time of an outbreak. Herpes is just a very small part of your world, albeit an annoying one at times. This is far from being trite or even obvious because one of the major problems with herpes is just that—having herpes continually plaguing your mind. It can become a vicious cycle that will contribute a great deal to your discomfort. So break the habit now. Focus outward on work, school, or fun and recreation.

Anxiety and worry about herpes increase physical discomfort and your perception of that discomfort. Reducing that anxiety takes your attention away from herpes for more productive purposes, and also reduces the experience of it. The links between physical discomfort and stress and anxiety are well established. When you have learned what you need to know about herpes from this book, you'll be able to drop most of the anxieties you may have developed about it and in so doing, reduce your discomfort accordingly.

Points to Remember
- ○ Unless really necessary, don't get in the habit of alleviating the discomfort with strong analgesic drugs.
- ○ Soothe the area by bathing or compresses, and then keep the area clean and dry.
- ○ Prevent as much chafing as possible.
- ○ Wear cotton underwear and loose clothing.
- ○ Work on ways to relieve tension and anxiety (see Chapter 9).
- ○ Establish your consistent personal regimen and then get on with whatever else you want to do in life.

3
Treatment of the Rash

Treatment of the rash itself has three aims:
- To keep viral activity to a minimum
- To prevent secondary bacterial infections
- To help your body's healing processes fight the virus and replace the rash with new tissue

This is the point at which we have to raise the question, "Where is the cure?" If there were a treatment effective in removing herpes virus from the body, there would be one line to this chapter. While there are many substances that will kill herpes virus, *none* can prevent recurrences. No substance yet developed can chase the virus into its nerve cell retreat or in any other way affect viral activity directly until the virus is outside the nerves in other tissue or fluid. Even then, as surface virus is being destroyed, more virus is entering the nerve cells to continue the process until the cycle is stopped.

With current technology, if we kill the virus in a nerve cell, we kill the cell. And nerve cells do not replace themselves as do other types of cells. Even so, killing the nerve cells harboring herpes is still no guarantee of killing all of the virus.

Current approaches are aimed at preventing virus production or destroying reactivated virus before a rash can develop. While none have yet made appreciable impact on recurrent herpes rashes, some success might be expected in the foreseeable future; five to ten years is a reasonable estimate (see Chapter 6). A solution to the larger problem of removal of the latent virus from the body is a very large scientific step and will take many years. Until then, the most effective treatment remains in your own body resources and in some helpful strategies. Since the virus production cycle does stop at some point during an outbreak and the rash disappears, then the mechanisms have to be in your own body. One of our jobs, as you will see, is to facilitate these as much as possible.

Don't chase new "cures" that pop up weekly in both credible and incredible sources written by professionals who should know better. Beware! When there is a treatment significantly more effective than your own body resources coupled with drying and cleaning the rash, it will quickly be available for everyone and will be well-known in the medical community. (See Chapter 6 for prescription substances—what they do and do not do. None of them provide cures despite their antiviral properties or immunological effects.)

When You Have a Rash

Keep the area clean and dry by washing with soap and water. *Cleaning* reduces the chances of secondary bacterial infections and *drying* kills surface virus and prevents a moist medium from developing, which can be helpful to the virus.

Bathing with Burow's solution or other drying salts will do the same thing and also soothe inflammation. Dabbing alcohol or ether on external sores will serve as an antiseptic. Some people find this helpful in the early stages of an outbreak. When sores have begun to heal, you may find this too abrasive on new tissue. Breaking the blisters with your hands, a pin, or needle is very risky. It can help spread the virus around, introduce a bacterial complication, or cause another abrasion.

Most antibacterial, anti-inflammatory, and other creams or ointments are not recommended. Though they can protect against other infections or reduce inflammation, their cream or oil base might actually provide a good medium for the virus to thrive. For example, Vaseline jelly would simply seal the area and protect the virus from drying, therefore, retarding healing.

Eat well and take a multivitamin supplement that includes B and C vitamins. Unless you have a specific nutritional or immunological deficiency and are under the care of a physician, don't take large doses of single vitamins. That will only benefit the profits of the producers and give your body something else to adjust to besides herpes.

Sleep well and don't do anything destructive to your body. Drinking too much alcohol will slow healing, as will too much coffee, too many cigarettes, and long, late evenings. *Relax*.

It is important to remember that physical or mental stress acts to deplete one's body resources. Reducing stress is a large topic which I will leave until Chapter 9. At this point, recognizing stressful tension as an enemy of fast healing is an important first step. Recognizing what specifically is stressful to you is a little more difficult.

The Placebo Effect

You'll notice I do not recommend any drug or nutritional substance to apply, inject or otherwise treat herpes rashes. However, I want to talk about something called the "placebo effect." Personal placebo routines can play an important role in adjustment and healing.

A placebo is officially an inert substance, sometimes in the form of a saline injection (water with salts added to make it compatible with body fluids) or a sugar pill, which has no direct physiological effect on a disease process. Placebos are often given to one group of people in a research study to provide a standard against which to compare the effects of a drug. A drug for a disease should be more successful in curing a disease than a placebo, or it would not be of much use as a specific antidote to the symptoms or cause of that disease!

The interesting fact is that in many cases where a particular illness is heavily laden with emotions or perceptions, the act of taking a placebo can in certain situations have a profound effect. This is particularly true with herpes because of its link with sexuality, a very personal and vulnerable part of a persons's life.

All new treatments "work!"—at least once, under the right conditions, just as a hypnotic suggestion will with the right person. Hope and excitement in a positive direction will definitely aid healing and prevent some outbreaks. But the stories of what "worked" for people and then somehow or other "stopped working" have become an epidemic in themselves. Jumping around among "cures" will certainly give you some success for some outbreaks because of the placebo effect, but they will work against you over the long haul. The tendency to always look for that one-shot annihilation of the virus is very strong, but later failures with new "cures" naturally cause disappointment and increase mistrust in other new treatments. It is often hard to admit to oneself that constantly trying new cures can set up a "negative" placebo effect, which in turn sets you up for failure, physically as well as mentally, and leaves you feeling more helpless and hopeless.

Instead, your goal is to establish a "positive placebo" routine through consistent application of the cleansing and soothing routines you have begun, and to learn how to take care of yourself during an outbreak. I use the term positive placebo because we seem to like labels in treating a condition, and the act of *doing something* or *taking something* in itself plays a role in adjustment. A good example of this is lysine, an over-the-counter amino acid supplement. Many people swear that lysine definitely is responsible for symptom reduction over time. While scientific studies show that it is no better than a placebo, it appears to provide part of the basis for adjustment for some people. It is the act of taking something, in this case something relatively harmless, that is important (see Chapter 6). Interestingly, when adjustment to herpes has occurred, cutting out the lysine seems to have no effect on symptoms!

Some touters of new "cures" will suggest a long-term regimen of treatment over several months. One case I came across involved the use of snake venom oil injections over two years! Another required acupuncture and diet change over eight to twelve months. I have nothing in particular against either snake venom oil or acupuncture, but whether such a physical treatment will work in your favor is questionable. However, it has been found that *any consistent program* that involves your playing an active role and in which you take care of yourself, living your life positively, will undoubtedly help adjustment by itself. These kinds of treatments may simply provide a vehicle or focus for that adjustment process, rather than having any direct impact on the herpes virus. Some of them may actually be quite harmful to you.

Points to Remember
○ Keep the rash clean and dry.
○ Use soap and water. Bathe in Burows solution to soothe and help dry the lesions.
○ Use alcohol to relieve itching and clean the rash.
○ Eat well, rest and slow down your daily routine.
○ Develop your treatment routine into a consistent regimen to begin as soon as an outbreak appears.

4
Contagion

By far the most important key to dealing with herpes is understanding and knowing what to do about contagion. Fears associated with being around other people, bearing or taking care of children, and, in general, being able to do and feel as you please, center on uncertainty about when or how you may be able to transmit the virus. This chapter is designed to give you the facts about contagion, elaborating on the information in Chapter 1, and showing you how contagion can be dealt with by exercising a minimum of care. This in turn will reduce your anxiety. When this issue is clear, you'll find that many other concerns you may have had will take care of themselves. Let's look at how herpes is transmitted, when a person is contagious, and what this means for you in terms of interacting with other people.

In my experience with men and women who have just contracted herpes, I've found that one run-through of the facts is not enough to allay fears and help the adjustment process get started. So I'll recap the facts already touched on and then go into them more fully.

Recognize that your first response to the potential risks may be much more alarming than is necessary, but it will serve the purpose of impressing you with the importance of preventative behavior that will ultimately free you to live with a minimum of disturbance in your routine and interpersonal relationships.

Transmission

Herpes can only be transmitted through **direct physical contact.** When the virus is in its latent stage, it is not transmissible. When there is sufficient virus present at the surface of the body, someone must touch it to become infected by it. The contagion area is highly localized and, so long as that area is not touched, transmission cannot occur. Oral-genital sex, if either a lip sore or genital sore is present, can result in transmission—lip to genitals or genitals to mouth. Herpes is highly contagious when sores are present.

The development of an active infection in another person depends on an interplay among:

○ how much virus invades that person's body through mucous membranes or a break in the skin.

○ whether or not the person has some measure of immunity to the virus.

○ his or her state of resistance to infection at that time.

Keep all these in mind as we work through what they mean for you.

I am assuming here that you have had a primary episode, and the virus has been dormant. A typical recurrence is preceded by some signs that the virus is becoming active in its nerve cell hideaway. These are the prodromal signs, or warning symptoms. Identify yours from the list in Chapter 9. They are not unlike symptoms you have felt before. These indicate viral activity and possible migration towards the body surface and may disappear without the appearance of a rash. This is very common once your body has adapted and you have some measure of control over recurrences. During prodromal periods, friction from intercourse or vigorous masturbation could bring on or facilitate an outbreak and rash if physical trauma is one of your particular trigger factors. Prodromal signs are a warning to be careful and think in terms of sex play other than active intercourse. The virus very rarely can be picked up on a swab at this time, but as you can see, you could play a role in speeding up the development of an outbreak. People often report breaking out the day after making love during the prodrome.

As soon as any signs appear on the skin, such as a red spot, you have to assume the presence of replicating virus. Culture tests are almost always positive at this point. If blisters develop, the fluid contained in them is very high in live virus. This is the time of the greatest risk. Even as the sores begin to heal and scab over, there is still action going on between your body and the virus, which you could aggravate by friction, increasing your chances of transmission. However, this is the turning point in an outbreak. Virus replication has stopped and the virus is beginning to recede from the body surface.

For a person who has had herpes for some time, presence of the virus in a recurrent outbreak (viral shedding) lasts on the average for the first three or four days in a typical seven-to-ten-day rash. So long as adjustment is going according to plan with nothing hindering it, reactivations should continue to decrease in severity. This is generally the common course, and you can, in all likelihood, get to the point of decreased severity in a reasonable time (see Chapter 9 on preventing recurrences).

First you must define your contagion parameters and plan your activities with them in mind. The conservative approach is to **assume the potential for transmission from just before sores show until the area is healed over with new skin.** There are times (at the beginning of an outbreak and during its healing) when it is not clear whether virus is present or not. The only way you could be absolutely sure when virus is present in an outbreak would be to have viral cultures taken at different stages. But this, of course, is not an accurate predictor for future outbreaks. So the safest approach is to exercise precautions from the time just before the rash shows until the scabs fall off and the area is covered with new skin.

There is some evidence that a previous history of herpes might offer some protection against subsequent infections. For instance, genital infections in someone with a history of cold sores will probably be less severe than in someone without. Similarly, subclinical infections may well offer some protection. But we have to be careful here. There are many varieties or strains of HSV I and II. While you may have partial protection, it is possible to get another infection in a different location. The reality, however, is that partners with herpes do not appear to give each other new infections in different locations very easily. Nonetheless, from what we know of the behavior of the virus, it is still possible.

The facts about infecting another person also apply to self-transfer. You can transfer herpes to another part of your own body. The eyes and fingers are particularly susceptible. This, in fact, doesn't happen very often with recurrent herpes. It is much more of a problem during a primary infection when the body has little or no defense against a viral invasion in another part of the body. Self-transfer from a genital infection to the eyes is virtually unknown, simply because of the location of the lesions though it is possible. It is more common from facial sores, but again, not very likely from recurrent outbreaks. You probably never will self-inoculate. If you take the precautions outlined later in the chapter, even the smallest risk should be removed.

Points to Remember
○ There is no virus in the skin between outbreaks.
○ Transmission can occur from just before sores show, encouraged by vigorous rubbing of the area, until new skin heals over the rash.
○ Your chances of developing a second genital infection from a partner or from self-inoculation are quite low, but nevertheless present.

How to Prevent Transmission

First, *know your own body and your characteristic symptoms during outbreaks.* Be obsessive about it at first so you won't have to be later on. Remember, you are building towards adjustment, control and ultimately freedom.

Second, *practice prevention and develop an automatic set of habits.* When you have an outbreak, do anything you like in your own life, or in relation to someone else's, *so long as the infected region is not touched directly.* Obviously, the most effective prevention then is abstinence from anything to do with that area. If you have a cold sore don't kiss anyone, anywhere, even in greeting, and especially don't kiss babies. Keep cold sores away from babies' reach at all times! If you have genital lesions, don't have intercourse. If you have either genital or oral lesions, do not engage in oral-genital lovemaking. There are many other ways to caress, fondle, and otherwise share intimacies.

I do recognize that there can be special problems both
for single people and for established couples in communicating easily about contagion. These will be discussed
in Chapter 8. The subject is not that difficult to deal with
but can be loaded with particular kinds of anxieties.

Will condoms help matters? The answer is yes and no:

○ A condom will help provide protection to a man against
low-level shedding of the virus from asymptomatic
women. This is a rare condition where a woman does not
experience symptoms while small amounts of the virus
may be present intermittently in cervical fluids.

○ A condom can only protect the areas covered. If a
man has sores which cannot be covered, then a condom will not be much use. The same thing holds if
a woman's lesions can contact areas not covered by
the condom.

○ There is a trade-off in using condoms even where
they do protect against lesion contact. You might
contribute to the spread of the virus, enlarging the
rash. Certainly you will aggravate the condition and
most likely retard healing.

Used wisely, condoms can help protect against herpes.
Used unwisely, there will either be no protection, or there
will be a trade-off in terms of healing and discomfort.

This brings us to the next question: "Can you be a
'carrier' of herpes without having symptoms?"

Nearly everyone in the United States will show antibodies to either HSV I or II by the age of fifty. This means
that they have been exposed to the virus at some time in
their lives. We can then assume that a great majority are
harboring herpes in the latent form, and in that sense are
"carriers." But, I repeat, *the latent virus cannot be transmitted to someone else.*

The real issue here is: "What are the chances of contracting herpes from someone who isn't aware of having
herpes or doesn't experience symptoms?" There is no

doubt that many people have herpes that has gone un-diagnosed because they have ignored symptoms or their symptoms were so mild as to not give sufficient cause for concern. Remember, the response to a herpes infection can range all the way from a subclinical infection up to a serious illness. In a subclinical infection, few or no identifiable signs may indicate inoculation by the virus; therefore, the person may be unaware of the condition. Subclinical infec-tions are probably quite common, and the future course of such an infection is difficult to predict. Identifiable recur-rences may or may not occur in the future. So we do have the possibility of what we called earlier "asymptomatic shedding of virus," or the potential for transmission when there are no obvious symptoms. It is impossible to de-termine if, in fact, asymptomatic shedding of virus is re-sponsible for any significant transmission of herpes, if any, since we do not know how much virus is necessary to in-teract with and break down the immune status of a person who is exposed.

You are continually being exposed to many kinds of infectious agents, either by choice or fortune, and your body fends them off very well, especially if it has had any prior experience with them. Only when these agents have a chance to avoid or beat body defenses does an infectious illness occur.

The most probable conclusion is that it is the people who are uninformed or who ignore or are careless about symptoms who are responsible for virtually all transmission of herpes (along with many other sexually transmitted dis-eases), and that transmission due to genuine asymptomatic viral shedding is extremely rare, if it occurs at all.

There is a flip side to this question that is much more bothersome emotionally for some people. It is the feeling of being potentially contagious all the time. This occurs in both men and women and often stands as a major hurdle to the free development of relationships—but it shouldn't! The feeling is really related to a kind of guilt before the fact: "What if I do infect someone even if I take all the precautions I think appropriate?" The word contamination often crops up here with a strong overlay of emotion that can be much more destructive than the realities of the risk of herpes transmission.

The fact is that couples informed about what symptoms to be aware of very rarely infect one another, and those that do are quite clear on how and when. If asymptomatic viral shedding were a significant contributor to transmission, many more people would be infecting their partners. From the clinical evidence this just doesn't seem to be the case! With mutual cooperation, the risk of transmission between partners should be essentially zero.

While there is reason for concern to take appropriate precautions against transmitting herpes, the elements of paranoia and fear tinged with guilt can serve to destroy intimacy and self-esteem much better than the herpes itself. It is hard to overstate this. Herpes can feed into the various ways we have been taught to think about ourselves, our bodies, and other people, and it can serve to undermine hard-won confidence. There is no reason for that. The emotional impact of herpes will be discussed more thoroughly in Chapter 7.

If you suffer from this constant feeling of contagion, it can help to have viral cultures taken to ease your mind. Use condoms, or use a spermicidal foam, which has antiviral properties, during intercourse. Letting this feeling stand in the way of close relationships is much more debilitating than herpes virus itself.

Toilet seats?

You will not get herpes from toilet seats, sample lipsticks at cosmetic counters or other inanimate objects. Unless the virus has an appropriate medium in which to survive, such as is deliberately provided in a culture laboratory, it dies quickly after leaving the body. When the virus dries, it dies. While water glasses, towels and tooth-brushes pose essentially no danger, to relieve anxiety, avoid sharing these while active sores are present.

The possibility of developing many kinds of infections through poor sanitary habits is always present, so it is good practice to avoid sharing personal toiletries when you have any kind of surface infection. (You have a human obligation to others.) Similarly, you should be especially careful about what, or who, you come into contact with if you have an open cut or sore in the skin. (You have a responsibility to yourself as well as to others.)

Some very young children have acquired genital herpes without "sexual" contact. The explanation for this is that the virus has been placed there by immediate transfer on a finger or towel from a facial sore that the baby has or a herpes sore that another person has, *not* from a towel that has been used some time before. As you know, babies are very active and very sexual. If a baby has facial herpes, be as careful as you can about the possibility of self-transfer by keeping the baby's hands off the sore.

The bottom line here, as in other areas of life, is that almost everything is possible—but the fact that it takes a lot of virus and direct contact with a mucous membrane or open skin abrasion to create a productive infection reduces the probability of contracting herpes from inanimate objects to essentially zero! *There has yet to be a case reported of herpes being caused in this way. Simple hygiene will relieve anxiety.*

Obsessive fear of the possibility of contracting herpes in this way is a much more serious pathology than having herpes.

Some Preventative Measures

○ Don't have genital intercourse when you or your partner have genital sores

○ Don't have oral sex when you or your partner have either oral or genital sores.

○ Use a condom when prodromal signs are present. The choice to use a condom when sores are present is yours to make after recognizing the risks to yourself and your partner. My advice is don't have intercourse at all when sores are present. Condoms will help protect against asymptomatic shedding.

○ When there are prodromal signs, avoid rough handling of the tissue around the rash area. If friction is a problem in general, use a lubricant such as K-Y jelly.

○ Don't poke and prod sores to check their progress.

If you have facial herpes look out for conscious or unconscious mannerisms which could spread the virus such as:

○ rubbing your chin;

○ licking a painful or itching part of your lip or covering it with saliva because it seems like a good idea;

○ playing with your moustache;

○ poking the sore with pens or pencils and then chewing on them;

○ smoking cigarettes in a way that you touch the sores;

○ running Chapstick over part or all of a fever blister and then over the rest of your lips.

After cleaning and drying, leave the rash alone, and have everyone else leave it alone, especially babies. There's no need for elaborate precautions as far as sleeping in bed with your partner is concerned. Wear cotton underwear over genital sores and avoid kissing with lip sores. Your partner will not pick up herpes from the pillows or bed sheets.

Wash your hands if they come in contact with the virus, especially first thing in the morning *before* you rub your eyes, or *before* inserting or removing contact lenses.

Never use saliva as the wetting agent whether or not you have herpes.

If you think you have been exposed to herpes, or if you have exposed anyone, take a shower and have them do likewise. Wash the area with soap and water.

Now, obviously, I'm again simply talking good hygiene, and a little obsessively at that. As I said earlier, this should become automatic habit very quickly, then the mental obsession can be dropped. The virus cannot penetrate undamaged skin, so don't be paranoid about it—just be careful. Exercise good normal hygiene and you will have no problem with either self-transfer, which is rare anyway, or transmission to partners.

How to Prevent Getting Herpes

After reading this chapter it should be fairly clear what measures you can take to help protect yourself from transmitting herpes. The information also can be used to protect yourself from getting herpes. I will spell it out so as there is no misunderstanding.

KNOW YOUR PARTNER. This is probably the most important point. Does your partner know what he or she is doing with your body, or your life? By the same token, do you know what you are doing with him or her? A little information goes a long way in making decisions about your well-being.

LOOK. If someone has a cold sore, stay away from it. As far as genital play is concerned, appearance of anything that shouldn't be there is always cause for concern. Now you don't need a microscopic examination to disrupt your whole evening. In normal sex play you can get a fair idea if anything is amiss without playing Sherlock Holmes. Take your time and play a little. Get to know your partner's body, which should be a pleasure in itself. Who wants to rush sex anyway?

ASK. One major problem in the spread of all sexually transmitted diseases is that the issue is hidden and laden with stigma, so freedom to exchange information about the most frequent human behavior is severely curtailed—a sorry state of affairs. If everyone knew the facts about genital herpes we would be a long way towards eliminating it in the population and drastically reducing its impact on individuals.

USE A CONDOM. With a new sex partner this is a good idea if you are at all unsure.

Your chance of contracting genital herpes is truly low if you exercise just a minimum of care.

5
Medical
Complications

In the last chapter, you saw that a series of "don'ts" can be turned into a set of natural habits that become automatic and let you adjust. Therefore, you don't have to worry so much. This also applies to the potential physical complications that you should be aware of. These may raise some initial concerns and rightly so. But again, the key is to first understand the issues and then put that knowledge to use. You then can drop much of the anxiety, since you'll know exactly what you'll have to be aware of and what you can do about it.

Secondary infections

The area of the herpes rash is very susceptible to secondary infection. If this does occur, healing will be retarded. In some cases a secondary infection may be more severe than herpes, so prevent this from happening. The rule of thumb is to follow the advice in Chapter 3. Keep the lesions clean and dry and leave them alone.

If you have a vaginal discharge or suspect that sores are not healing the way they should, see your physician to make sure that a secondary infection is not complicating the healing process. Do not self-medicate with whatever you might have in your medicine chest. Get correct diagnosis and treatment. This is very important. Remember, over-the-counter and prescription antibacterial, antiseptic, and anti-inflammatory creams and ointments generally are *not* recommended.

Herpes of the eye (herpes keratitis)

A potentially much more serious problem is that of getting herpes in the eye. The cornea of the eye, the outer transparent covering of the iris, is particularly vulnerable to herpes infections. (There are 20,000 new cases of blindness caused by herpes per year.) While the eye can be the primary site of infection, in adults, herpes keratitis is often caused by transfer of the virus from an open primary facial infection. Remember, a primary infection is a first-time infection. If you have a primary infection, get a physician's help and keep the infection clean and dry. In the case of cold sores, keep them away from children, especially their eyes.

WHAT TO DO ABOUT HERPES KERATITIS. The chances of developing an eye infection by self-transfer from recurrent infections as opposed to primary ones are very small. But let's remove even this small chance with simple and obvious precautions.

First, be aware of any ways in which you may touch active sores. Then observe the rules of good hygiene. It's always tempting to check the progress of a new sore, even when it hasn't developed yet, by poking and prodding. Don't! You could pick up the virus and transfer it inadvertently to your eye.

If you are concerned that your eye has become infected see a physician immediately. Symptoms appear about two to ten days after contact and show first as irritation or pain, or a feeling of something in the eye. There will be a sensitivity to light and perhaps blurring in the visual field. As the infection progresses, the eye will become red and swollen with tearing. As with herpes in other areas, the attack will clear up and the virus will become dormant, possibly to recur in the future. Again, do not wait for this to occur. The danger of not getting treatment is that permanent scarring of the infected area can occur and cause loss of vision. However, the good news is that diagnosis of herpes of the eye is relatively easy and, unlike recurrent genital or facial herpes, there are quite a few very effective treatments that can quickly stop and remove the active infection.

Remember: Self-inoculation of the eye is very uncommon from recurrent infections in the genital area. But worrying about it now simply will help you form good hygiene habits. Then you can stop worrying.

Herpes and Cervical Cancer

There is an association between genital herpes and cancer of the cervix in women. This might sound very alarming as a cold statement, but it actually isn't when you understand the facts and exactly what to do about them.

First, cancers are caused by a multitude of interacting factors. Having genital herpes does not mean that a woman will necessarily develop cervical cancer. What the scientific evidence does tell us is that the risk of developing cervical cancer is greater by a factor of somewhere between five and eight times in women who have had genital herpes. However, it is important to note that the factors that provide the greatest risks toward cervical cancer are age at first intercourse (the younger the greater the risk) and the number of sexual partners (the more partners, especially uncircumcised partners, the higher the chances). The relationships here are very complex. Pinpointing real and specific causative agents for cervical cancer has proved to be very difficult. But what you should understand is that herpes is one agent among many that increases the risk.

WHAT TO DO ABOUT MONITORING CERVICAL CANCER. Fortunately, it is fairly easy to monitor the potential for cervical cancer and to deal with problems, should they arise. Establish a good and open relationship with your gynecologist and remind him or her of your herpes history. Make sure you **have a Pap test every six months,** which checks the cells in the cervix and detects abnormalities. When changes are detected early, the treatment is simple and virtually 100 percent effective. Bear in mind that the majority of abnormalities that show up in Pap examinations are not indicators of cancerous conditions. But by having routine tests you are protecting yourself from the future development of unnecessary complications.

Herpes and Pregnancy

If you have facial herpes, pregnancy intrinsically is not a problem. But don't expose a newborn infant to facial sores. Just exercise the precautions already discussed. If you have recurrent genital herpes, your major concern is that the baby may pick up the virus by contact during passage through the birth canal at the time of delivery. Infections of the fetus in the womb have been reported. These are very rare and only occur from primary infections acquired during pregnancy where, as you'll remember, the virus has free play in the body until antibodies develop to drive the virus into latency. In come primary infections, the virus manages to be transported by the bloodstream across the placental barrier to infect the fetus. This does not occur with recurrent herpes! Recurrent genital herpes is highly localized. The dormant virus does not work its way up the birth canal to cross the placenta.

The figures on infants contracting herpes during delivery range from around 300 to 1500 newborns out of 3 to 3.5 million live births per year. However, with proper monitoring and precautionary measures, it is theoretically possible to prevent all of these. Tragically, not everyone is aware of how to do this. I say tragically because a herpes infection to the newborn can be very serious indeed. The virus can quickly take over essentially defenseless tissue, resulting in death of the infant in more than half the cases and severe brain damage in many of the remainder. After about 3 months, the baby is much more able to recover from a herpes invasion, and the crucial danger period is over.

Does this mean an automatic Caesarean delivery for every woman who has herpes? Absolutely not. So long as herpes is not present in the birth canal at the time of delivery, everything should proceed as normal for a vaginal delivery. If herpes is present then, a Caesarean section is the appropriate way to protect the baby.

WHAT TO DO ABOUT HERPES AND PREGNANCY. First, work closely with your obstetrician. He or she must know about your history with herpes. You should both start to be able to identify, as accurately as possible, the particular characteristics of your outbreaks—prodromal signs, site or recurrence, healing time, and so on. You should be fairly good at this by the time you have put into effect the advice in Chapter 8. Then the doctor will be in a better position to help and advise you.

Recurrences during the pregnancy should be no

cause for concern in and of themselves so long as everything else is fine. As you near term, you will be
monitored more closely to identify if herpes is present or
not. This will mean more frequent examinations and viral culture tests. A decision will then be made as to the
best way to proceed. If there are signs of a recurrence
near term which could interfere with delivery, a
Caeserean birth will be recommended. If everything is
clear and well, this will not be necessary. The whole secret is a close monitoring of the state of the birth canal all
the way through the pregnancy and especially near the
time of delivery.

> Points to Remember
> ○ Give your obstetrician all available in-
>   formation
> ○ Work closely with him or her, and there
>   should be no danger to your baby. If
>   every expectant mother who has genital
>   herpes were monitored, there would be
>   no danger from herpes for any baby.

Can you nurse your baby? By all means. Just don't let
the baby come in contact with herpes sores in any way. Wash
your hands as you normally would before nursing and exercise your hygiene precautions. Thousands of healthy babies
are born every year to mothers who have genital herpes.

The potential complications such as secondary infections, herpes of the eye, cervical cancer, and complications
during birth can be quite frightening to people. But in fact,
they can all be dealt with fairly easily with some simple precautions. Getting over the fear is the worst part, and all it
takes is accurate information.

6
Medical
Treatments

While there are some promising substances being investigated that can interfere with or kill the herpes virus, none are able to eradicate it from the body after it has been able to move into a latent state. So the potential for reactivation after treatment is always there. There is therefore no outright cure unless all the virus can be killed off during a *primary* infection.

It may be possible to get rid of all or most of the virus before the latent phase can begin, in which case the potential for recurrence could be removed or at least reduced. While possible, it is unlikely, since it takes a few days for symptoms to show after exposure. By then, the virus has had free play in the body for that period of time.

The largest impact can be obtained with a treatment during this primary episode. Once recurrences have developed it is a different story. The chance of eradicating herpes from its dormant state is essentially zero. Hence, there is no "one-shot" cure.

Medical treatments for recurrences have taken several directions:

- To kill or interfere with the virus after reactivation has begun.
- To set up conditions in the body in a more general way, that may help keep the virus dormant;
- Doing something to the body that helps natural healing processes and so shortens outbreaks.

There is no "one-bullet" cure because nothing has been developed that can go in and snip the virus manufacturing source from its latent retreat.

There are very effective treatments for the control of ocular herpes (of the eyes) and herpes reactivations suffered by people undergoing immune-suppressing treatment (for cancer or organ transplant rejection) that severely reduces normal immune responses to infection. These are of immense importance for organ-transplant recipients and cancer patients, but have little direct relevance to the day-to-day problems of recurrent genital herpes. There are, however, several substances which in some cases have apparently achieved the aims of reducing frequency and duration of recurrences. This is a complicated issue with many factors involved in the mechanisms of virus reactivation and replication. We will run through the major treatments and the rationales behind them with the goal of understanding what is true and untrue about them so that you won't hurt yourself physically with misapplication of substances, you won't chase cures indiscriminately, and you won't worry about missing out on some "new cure."

Antiviral Agents

Antiviral agents serve to interfere in some way with virus production and thus are aimed at stopping the action of the virus in disrupting surface tissue and causing the rash.

Antiviral technology is the great new breakthrough in the world of infectious diseases in general. Herpes, however, is a more difficult virus to catch than most because of its latency factor. The list of products to help herpes includes the following:

ZOVIRAX (acyclovir). Approved by the Food and Drug Administration in March, a good antiviral ointment very useful in initial infections and for immune-compromised patients. Acyclovir in large quantities has been proven effective in control of the very serious herpes reactivations that can occur in these patients. The treatment regimen is not appropriate to ordinary cases of recurrent herpes since it often involves intravenous or continual application that can only be provided in supervised settings. The evidence from its use with recurrent genital herpes suggests that it might reduce viral shedding time by about one day during a recurrence. The manufacturers are now promoting a series array of clinical tests to see if it might further reduce viral shedding if applied early enough in an outbreak. The rationale is that if all the virus is caught as it is coming out of its dormant state, an outbreak may be aborted, or at least curtailed. There's no way to know this yet. Reducing viral shedding by one day doesn't help very much, since a rash is still present and it is impossible to tell when viral shedding has stopped without culture tests. Reducing the length of time that the rash is present is really what we're after. Again, acyclovir cannot attack the dormant virus and so cannot prevent recurrences in and of itself. But at the moment, it appears that Zovirax might be one of those things to have on hand when an outbreak shows up, perhaps to supplement cleaning and drying. I expect it will help some people for a while. Its long-term effect cannot be predicted since it cannot affect latency. Whether or not its use might contribute to speeding the adaptation process is another question that requires further research. Experimentation presently is being done to develop an oral version of the drug.

STOXIL. The brand name for a compound containing the antiviral idoxuridine (IDU). It has been useful in ocular herpes but has no apparent effect on the course and frequency of genital outbreaks.

ARA-A (adenine arabinoside or vidaribine). This is highly successful with ocular herpes and herpes encephalitis, but ineffective on the course and frequency of genital outbreaks.

Both Stoxil and Ara-A can have undesirable toxic side effects when used in doses that may have any useful impact on genital recurrences.

2 DEOXY-D-GLUCOSE (2DG). Licensed for experimentation only and not for general release, shows some promise especially for initial infections. It is a good antiviral, and there doesn't seem to be any problem with toxicity. It has had some success in a select group of women with severe symptoms. The factors responsible are unknown. It serves as a great viral inhibitor when it can get at the virus, but again is unlikely to do anything with the latent phase.

VIRAZOLE (ribavirin). Available only outside of the U.S. There is no evidence that this substance is better than any other compound.

INTERFERON. One of the great new hopes in many areas of viral work. But there is as yet no evidence to suggest a beneficial effect with recurrent herpes. Interferon is manufactured by the body's own cells. It may be more productive to help your body in the direction of producing its own interferon by good health behavior than to apply it from the outside!

These antiviral drugs have evolved from a growing body of antiviral research that is also providing insight into the herpes viruses in general. They can kill viruses, or prevent their replication to some degree, but cannot prevent recurrences. Even with their application, a host of factors operate in recurrences to affect how long outbreaks last. Invariably, adaptation takes place over time with or without particular antivirals and recurrences become fewer and shorter. The antiviral research is helping to illuminate the reasons for this, but the ability to remove the latent virus is still some way off.

Antibiotics

Penicillin or tetracycline have no effect on herpes virus. They are antibacterial, not antiviral. Despite this, a version of Trobicin (spectimomycin) has just been patented as a herpes treatment. May the buyer beware! Consult a physician for guidance through the pharmaceutical compendium.

Corticosteroids, Liquid Nitrogen Freezing, and Povidone Iodine (Sold as Betadine)

These have no proven effects. Corticosteroid creams and ointments that operate as anti-inflammatory agents are, in general, not recommended by physicians and scientists involved in herpes work, since they may actually delay healing and ultimately work against body adjustment.

Immune System Modulation

Another method is to manipulate or modulate immune responses, or help the body's immune mechanisms in a more general way so that viruses are swept up quickly and recurrences shortened. In cases where immune deficiencies are present, such manipulation may indeed make people healthier. But this is an area requiring specific diagnosis, not the random application of immune modulating drugs in otherwise healthy people. Also, there are several pitfalls. Manipulating immune response with a drug to exactly the correct level is difficult and harrowing. If you stimulate immune responses too far, sometimes the result is to reverse beneficial effects into detrimental ones.

BCG (Bacillus Calmette-Guerin). This is a bacteria vaccine against TB. It helps in a general way to increase the immune response but has no specific effect on herpes.

SMALLPOX, POLIO AND INFLUENZA VACCINES. These have the same rationale—to increase the immune response in general. They don't prevent recurrences nor shorten outbreaks.

VACCINATION with live herpes virus or inactivated herpes virus. This (Lupidon G or Lupidon H in the latter case) is doomed to failure. Since having the virus itself in a latent form doesn't protect against herpes, then vaccination won't have any beneficial effect either.

INOSIPLEX OR METHISOPRINOL (Isoprinisine), LEVAMISOLE, TYMOSIN (Thymus extract). These all have immune system modulation properties and all have no direct effect on herpes reactivation, but they may help immune responses after the virus is activated. However, the significance of this is small where the immune response of an individual is within normal limits. They may have an effect on primary herpes where immune defenses are often stretched to their limit.

In any case, you are playing around with well-controlled natural body processes. Unless there is evidence that indicates serious problems with immune responses (outside of those caused by chronic stress, which can severely depress them), these substances will have limited or no effect in nearly all cases of herpes.

Other Treatments

LITHIUM. This is a potent psychoactive substance used for depression-related psychiatric disorders, that cannot really be considered. It is true that clinical work with Lithium and depression has shown that often when a depression is lifted, herpes symptoms are reduced. But curing a depression is more effective for herpes than use of Lithium itself.

DYE-LIGHT TREATMENTS. This is the application of a dye to the rash with exposure to ultraviolet light. These can be dangerous by creating mutants of the virus that may become carcinogenic in certain situations. Stay away from this type of treatment.

LASER TREATMENTS. This is a new technology that destroys herpes infected tissue with laser beams. It is still in its infancy, and again there is no evidence that it has anything to do with preventing recurrences. It may be helpful in primary cases.

DMSO (diamethyl sulfoxide). This is simply a "carrier" which can help other substances, good or bad, deeper into body tissues. Its value in transporting other compounds to act against herpes has not shown any significance. In itself it will do nothing and may be dangerous in high doses.

AMP (ADENOSINE 5-MONOPHOS-PHATE). A natural occurring substance, AMP plays a major role in cell response and metabolism. Some people with fairly severe herpes infections have been found to have low blood levels of this compound. Restoring this to normal may be the mechanism whereby AMP has helped some people. There is currently no way to know if use of AMP has any effect in other cases. Again, natural body adjustment should take care of lowered AMP levels and do a better job in the long run than an injection program. AMP does seem as if it may be of immediate usefulness in tough cases. But the proper tests have not been carried out, and the long-range effects are unknown. The role of placebo cannot be ruled out.

HERPIGON (zinc sulphate). This compound may have some antiviral properties, but like the other antivirals it can't touch recurrences and doesn't live up to its name.

ETHER, ALCOHOL, AND ACETONE. These are all solvents that will dry lesions and kill the virus. They, especially ether, will sting or burn on sensitive tissue. While there is no reason to suppose they will shorten outbreaks, they will help keep the area free from secondary infections and will dry sores to inhibit viral spread. Alcohol is also very cheap.

SPERMICIDAL FOAMS. Nonoxynol-9 is a common ingredient in contraceptive foams that appears to have antiviral properties. It may give some protection from low-level viral shedding.

DIETARY AGENTS. In general, dietary requirements are related to changes in body processes under different conditions. Attacking herpes in an otherwise healthy body with large doses of single nutrients such as vitamins C, E, A or minerals like magnesium or zinc, amino acids, etc. will have little or no effect. However, conditions such as chronic stress or unusual dietary habits can result in deficiencies that can affect immune system functioning and cellular repair. Correcting deficiencies is really what we are interested in here rather than making additions to good general nutrition. There can, in fact, be a danger of operating in favor of the virus with massive doses of single nutrients. For example, vitamin E is a fine substance that can enhance general resistance to infection. But megadoses can serve to inhibit many immune responses. A good multivitamin nutritional backup is a good idea. But anything else should be used only after a consultation with your physician.

LYSINE. A single amino acid that has received considerable attention because it is cheap and readily available, lysine is reported to inhibit viral growth by blocking the use of another amino acid, argenine, in virus manufacture. The ratio of lysine to argenine has been shown to be a factor in virus production *in vitro* (outside the body in a laboratory). Lysine and argenine are essential to many body reactions and are found in large quantities in normal balanced diets—lysine in red meat, potatoes, brewers yeast and milk, and argenine in chocolate, nuts and raw cereals. There are no definitive results showing that altering the lysine/argenine balance has any effect on recurrences even though subjective reports from thousands of herpes sufferers appear to support the notion that lysine supplements help to reduce symptoms. There is no clinical proof of this. Lysine may be labelled as a great placebo.

The picture that emerges from exploring the medical-treatment pharmacopoeia:

○ *Antivirals and associated research are providing optimism for the future.* Large strides have been made in the treatment of ocular herpes, encephalitis, and herpes in immune-compromised patients. No substance can be said to prevent outbreaks of genital or facial herpes directly, although some individuals have been helped. Viral shedding may be reduced, but this is minimal help, since the rash is still there.

○ *Playing with vaccines and other immune modulators doesn't appear to be a good idea, according to our current knowledge, or lack of it.* Checking for deficiencies in immune function in cases that are more severe than they should be may be a useful avenue. These cases, however, are often linked to chronic stress. Removing the stress most often brings immune responses back to normal, with automatically reduced herpes symptoms.

○ *Dietary approaches are also less than helpful.* Additions to a normal diet will most likely do nothing against herpes, while corrections of diet problems may well have an effect.

In essence, while a few substances may help the body fight herpes, none can eradicate the recurrent virus.

7
Personal Problems

There are certain personal problems that often accompany herpes, but you either can avoid them or deal with them fairly easily if they arise. Whether you have herpes, have a likelihood of contracting it in the future, or are associated with people who do get herpes recurrences there are some important points you should be aware of.

You must remember that what the whole process comes down to is a process of adjustment—a physical adaptation over time and an emotional adjustment to living with the possibility of occasional disruptions in sexual freedom and spontaneity. And that's all.

Individuals with herpes fall into three main categories and have distinct emotional responses. First are those who develop a recurrent infection with effects so minor as to scarcely affect their personal life at all, and whose main problem is occasional concern about prevention. These people form the largest group by far. The fact that most people have been exposed to HSV I (on the face) but don't have any kind of serious problem associated with it is a good indicator of what happens with most genital herpes infections as well. Depending on the interaction between virus load, resistance, immunity and type of person, after the primary infection, symptoms are few and minor. Of course, an important adjunct to this is that there may be many people spreading herpes because they "have these little red marks once in a while which are no big deal." A little public education here would do an awful lot of good.

Then there are those who develop recurrences and who, with good information and counseling, take appropriate precautions, adjust their life-styles accordingly, and experience a minimum of disruption in their daily lives.

Lastly are those who have recurrences that affect their life-styles and freedom more seriously and increase their fears and anxieties in such a way as to present real and sometimes severe difficulties in adjustment.

This chapter is written primarily for the third group, while it will educate the public at large about these personal issues.

Apart from the potential for physical complications, the major problem with herpes isn't so much in the virus itself, but in the ways its presence can create fears, doubts and disruptions in day-to-day living and planning, particularly in interpersonal relationships. Fortunately, these effects can be reduced significantly, even in cases where the initial impact of contracting herpes and contemplating recurrences is serious and difficult.

Herpes can cause problems in several ways. Fears

about contagion, childbirth and physical complications are rational and are not to be dismissed too lightly. They can, however, as you have seen in the preceding chapters, be addressed rationally and dealt with. Unfortunately, the media has managed to fuel these fears to exaggerated proportions. Sensational headlines like "Sex makes you sick" in the now defunct New York *Soho News,* and "Herpes: The New Sexual Leprosy" in *Time* magazine may make great press, but they also instill needless fear in people who have not contracted genital herpes, and murderous rage in some of those who have! These kinds of stories tend to stir up and prolong anxieties about interpersonal difficulties, when in fact such difficulties can be managed and dealt with quite efficiently.

Lack of good information is also a culprit, as is the way in which information is presented to people. What is important is a recognition that the notion of "recurrent" carries with it an automatic need for good usable information to alleviate understandable concerns about intimacy with others. Emotional responses to the facts of herpes are very natural and must be put in the right perspective when information about herpes is presented. While we deal with some of the more serious side effects of herpes that you may run into, keep in mind that we are working always towards positive, fulfilling interpersonal success.

The emotional reactions to herpes can range all the way from feeling isolated, withdrawing from others; becoming obsessed with herpes; feeling that herpes will invade all areas of your life; feeling embarrassed, guilty or shameful; to becoming depressed through feeling helpless, thinking that relationships will be difficult, if not impossible, or that people will reject you.

It is natural that you should experience some or all of these feelings at one time or another, but unnatural if they persist for too long. However, that should not have to be the case, and won't be if the feelings can be acknowledged and dealt with directly.

Herpes and Interpersonal Fears

Since genital herpes, by definition and nature, is an infection associated with sexuality, it often becomes thought of as a sexual disease, or a disease of sexuality, rather than a rash that occurs on the sexual organs. Notice the distinction. Your means of expression of sexuality can sometimes be affected, but not your sexuality per se. Unfortunately, these two ideas are sometimes difficult to keep separate, and a syndrome of emotional responses can develop. Thoughts about contagion can lead in two directions—the first to a pervasive and continual fear of spreading herpes; and the second to thoughts that one's sexuality in general has been irrevocably damaged. These in turn can lead to a series of feelings much worse than the virus and to behavior reinforcing the bad feelings in a vicious cycle.

A large part of this problem stems from societal training—that sex and sexuality are to be dealt with differently, as well as with more secrecy, than other parts of our lives. Men with herpes more often worry about performance—also an idea fed by cultural orientation.

You might be thinking, herpes has damaged my sexuality. Therefore I am not the same as I was, which makes me feel bad about myself. This gives me problems in dealing with other people and prevents me from getting close to them. I am now less free than before because I feel worse about myself. So I am withdrawn because my sexuality is damaged, because I have herpes.

Notice the circularity.

You may indeed experience associated feelings of embarrassment, shame, or even guilt followed by social withdrawal. Some people develop a fear of rejection because herpes has eroded their feelings of attractiveness, desirability, and self-esteem. Others go through periods of depression and helplessness, or read the medical literature avidly, becoming experts on the details of biochemistry, immunology, virology and several other "-ologies," with the same result—the energy expended only leading to more disappointment, frustration, and worry.

Sexual and social dysfunctions can occur as a direct result of the emotional impact of herpes. I want it to be clear that feelings of depression, of helplessness, and of loss of freedom and dreams can be very natural reactions. These are emotional responses to the myths, fears, and social stigmas associated with herpes. But these effects are also common responses to other recurrent or chronic physical conditions or to life's problems in general, which can seem insurmountable until understood and addressed. The crucial dimension of genital herpes that distinguishes it from other disorders is that it is associated with sexuality.

Even the most well-adjusted and psychologically attuned men and women are not immune to part or all of this emotional syndrome. There are all sorts of social and cultural reasons for the interplay between the physical and psychological aspects of a disease like herpes, especially since herpes is often contracted during the periods in a person's life when he or she is experimenting with sexual feelings. One tends to think in terms of outright cures for the physical aspects of the virus, and the less concrete problem of the personal aspects can get hidden and lost in the drug technology and search for a cure. So your job is to identify your emotional feelings, deal with them, and get on with the business of living as quickly, rationally, and skillfully as possible.

Some Common Feelings

Herpes virus does not cause impotence, sterility, or neurological deficiency, although it may cause discomfort during or before recurrences! But it's quite possible that it may affect your emotions and cause transient impotence or lack of desire.

Herpes has the great capacity to tap into and feed on other concerns and emotional styles that people have. While concern about contagion is an important emotional response, guilt is a useless one as it is in most other situations. Feelings that you are being punished justly or unjustly are not only unproductive, but downright undermining. Guilt comes from many sources in our culture and getting herpes can often reactivate other guilt feelings about bodies, behavior, and so forth.

Feelings of being contaminated all the time stem from the same roots. Since you now know what to do about contagion, you need not feel that way. ***Separate herpes and your relationship with herpes from other areas of your life.***

Anger is natural and needs to be let out, but not on yourself! This only leads to self-dislike and more anger. Cure-chasing invariably leads either to more disappointment and frustration, or to more anger and depression. The anger about herpes subsides automatically in direct proportion to your adjustment and capacities to coexist with and control herpes as a life disrupter. But by all means be angry. You're quite right in feeling that more research is needed to find a cure for herpes (see resources section for an outlet for this). And you are probably quite right in being angry about other circumstances related to herpes. But for now, harness that great motivator towards any of the challenges that getting herpes may have set up.

Fear of rejection is very common because herpes can initially deflate your sexual ego. Some people's self-worth revolves entirely around their sexuality. For them, this can be a tough problem to deal with, but it shouldn't be for two good reasons. First, you now know a great deal about contagion and how to combat it, and you know that you can do pretty much what your heart desires between outbreaks. In fact you can do a great deal during them too (in the way of intimacy), if you exercise a little care and creativity.

If you are single, the fear associated with herpes can play even more tricks on you. In part, this fear is based on a person feeling incomplete, not whole, or on anxiety that he or she won't be able to perform properly, or at the right time.

Despite the current fashion for "relating" and "communicating," real intimacy in talking about needs and desires is still difficult for many people. First time sex or sex between people who do not yet know one another very well is rarely anxiety-free; one or both persons usually have something on the line. It usually involves performance and other forms of expectations and often leaves out ease, good feelings, and plain interactive passion. Hence, in someone who has herpes, performance anxiety, although totally unrelated to herpes, can feed upon this additional fear and anxiety that herpes creates.

What about somebody else having to deal with your having herpes? You may feel like nobody's going to want to nurse you, or sleep with you, or deal with you when you have herpes. Nobody's going to need to nurse you and, in fact, you won't have to nurse yourself much either once you've adjusted to herpes. A little understanding, comfort, and encouragement is part of what friends and lovers can provide, and it is not too much to expect. If you can't have some of that in a relationship, there's something wrong with your choice of partner.

The initial talking through with a potential long-term partner is the psychological hurdle you have to clear (and in the next chapter we'll discuss exactly how to do this). Then many other things will fall into place. Disappointments from rejections have occurred, of course, as they occur in other circumstances in life as well. However, there is a tendency to withdraw from the possibility of rejection (I've seen this happen both in long-standing relationships and in first meetings of people drawn to each other), or to set things up so as to drive the other person away—

not uncommon without herpes as an issue! From all my experience in treating men and women who contract herpes, it is clear that the issue of communicating that they have herpes is viewed as the most difficult stage in adjustment—mostly because of fear of rejection. But my experience has also shown that this can usually be overcome successfully and quickly.

I've come across rejections blamed on herpes where it was not the culprit, or relationship breakups where one or the other partner had herpes and where, again, herpes was not the reason, although sometimes a ready scapegoat. But I have not seen herpes, *per se*, break up a relationship or prevent one from developing, except in some special cases with extreme symptoms.

The people who do run into personal and emotional difficulties come through them. They make, break, and maintain relationships, sexual and otherwise, and live with vigor, free from depression and self-doubt associated with herpes.

The real danger lies in letting the emotional syndrome become more powerful and recurrent than the rash itself.

8
Discussing Herpes with Partners and Friends

Since herpes is bound to bother you in some physical or emotional way, you won't be able to hide it forever —it will come up at some point in your interactions with others. On those occasions where you want to encourage more lasting relationships than casual encounters, it is important to be able to discuss herpes in the least threatening manner possible. While there is no best way to talk about herpes, there are better ways. Fit the guidelines and strategies presented in this chapter into your own personal style.

Here's how to prepare to talk about herpes to a prospective partner. You should know the physical symptoms and their antidotes discussed in Chapters 1 through 5. Remember especially that the problems of contagion and physical complications can all be dealt with fairly easily. We know from clinical information that most informed people do not transmit herpes to their partners within relationships. The problem of herpes transmission in general is primarily one of ignorance and carelessness. With informed participation and mutual cooperation, the chance of transmitting herpes to a partner is extremely small.

You should be in reasonable control of herpes in your life, in touch with how you feel about yourself and your relationship with herpes. By now you know your own patterns and have established ways of dealing with your own physical problems. Those accomplishments will come across when you talk with other people. Don't deny that herpes can be a damned nuisance that can restrict your freedom at times—so can other things, such as your work and your moods.

You are *not* a *herpetic!* In fact, that word should not have been invented. Herpes is just a very small part of who you are.

Now ask yourself how you usually talk to other people about things that are important to you. Don't change your style now unless it hasn't worked for you in the past. Is your usual style one that sets you up for rejection? Some people naturally do just that and the social stigma of herpes can exaggerate that tendency. You can avoid that particular trap.

You should recognize that the first time you have sex with someone you will be feeling some anxiety that has nothing to do with herpes. So don't worry about performance. Just feel comfortable with the person, because your ego isn't entirely in your sex organs. Also remember that herpes causes only occasional sexual limitations.

Get to know the person, at least a little. This isn't a speech about morality. Just develop a sense of how your partner responds to your needs and possible quirks and how you reciprocate. In other words, develop a little intuitive trust.

How and when should you discuss herpes? Choose a time and a place when you will be comfortable answering detailed and perhaps personal questions. A quiet time at home or perhaps during a walk might be good. During a cocktail party or just when you have begun to make love are definitely not good times.

Be careful not to let your other needs for approval, affection, or personal validation get in your way. Take charge of the situation and plan ahead. Rehearse with your friends. This will help to give you confidence and allow for feedback about you and your relationship with the other person. This can be very valuable information. Talking things over doesn't cure viruses, but it does cure a lot of vague emotional distortion and hidden anxieties.

Now that you have prepared for success, find an appropriate time and situation and simply broach the subject calmly and directly. You don't have to raise the issue first thing after meeting someone you like. Since some people tend to judge others by hard and fast preconceived notions, you may want to wait a bit. If you bring up the subject too soon, it could be seen as presumptuous (you are assuming imminent lovemaking). Or it may fit the cliche that if you reveal the worst things about yourself to someone and are still accepted, then that person really must care and you are safe. That's not really a very effective way to win friends, influence people, or establish a relationship.

A not untypical case illustrates many of the dilemmas associated with telling others about herpes. Dan (not his real name) fell into the trap of setting himself up for rejection despite the best intention in the world. He contracted herpes from a casual affair after a party but was adamant that the virus would not rule his life. Dan "solved" the problem of recurrences by choosing not to tell anyone, and arranged dates only when he was symptom-free. This worked to keep herpes out of his private life for a year and a half, and nobody knew the difference. But the deception began to depress him, and he really wanted to settle down a bit.

He met someone he was unusually attracted to, had lunch with her, and decided it was time to cross the bridge he had been avoiding. At their first dinner date, Dan announced, in his usual forthright manner, "I know you like me, but I have a secret to tell you that's been bothering me since we met. I have herpes, and I thought you should know about it right away. Now I don't want you to get worried, it's not a big deal. I'm just telling you so there is no misunderstanding. I want to be straight with you because if we get to know each other better, you'll have to deal with it."

Not surprisingly, Mary (also a pseudonym) was rather alarmed and somewhat confused.

Dan could probably have saved the situation at this point after his openers (it would have been difficult, but possible) had he been able to demonstrate that he could handle herpes responsibly without passing on a large measure of its burden to his new friend. But as often happens during such an explanation, he got quite carried away with his helplessness and particularly his anger at "the damned doctors and researchers" and the girl who gave him herpes.

Mary really sympathized. It was obvious to Dan that she felt for him, for this terrible thing that had happened to him. But the game was lost by this time. While very nice about it, Mary really didn't want to take on the burdens that Dan had presented to her, and not unexpectedly, she politely rejected him on the telephone later in the week.

Can you see what was going on?

Dan, in keeping with his personality and way of handling himself, played it very straight. He was certainly quite honest. In this case, his history is telling. Dan had broken

9
Preventing
Recurrences

This chapter will provide the information you need in order to control recurrences and the effects of recurrences to as high a degree as possible. Not only can you gain some measure of control through knowing your own body and anticipating problem situations, but you will also be able to work towards reduced frequency and duration of outbreaks.

In most cases, herpes seems just to "go away" (become essentially dormant) in a few years. For many, this disappearance occurs much more rapidly; for others, the adaptation process is less successful. Nothing just goes away by itself! Something happens to cause diminished symptoms. But you can play a large role in the process of reducing symptoms to their physiological minimum, which is permanent or close to permanent dormancy.

The focus will be on three main areas: general health and well-being; the prodromal and trigger mechanisms for recurrences and how you can eliminate some and use others to your benefit; and finally, stress, that blanket category for a host of factors that influence recurrences, recovery, and adaptation in general.

The effects of herpes symptoms on the emotional and behavioral areas of life is quite clear from Chapter 8. This also occurs in the opposite direction to a large degree. Things you do, think, and feel often can take on the capacity to feed back into the physical aspects of the problem. This channeling of life issues into symptoms is, at least for a while, very common. It's as if herpes becomes the path of least resistance for stresses of the world until that link is broken. This section should help alleviate that problem and the information will be applicable to the many areas of your life that can be touched by herpes.

General Physical Well-being

Eat well, sleep well, exercise properly, and behave with your body's best interests in mind. You can consult your physician or a good book on diet for nutritious and balanced eating habits. But be careful. There are as many myths around what is good and bad for you in the way of food as there are about herpes. A normal well-balanced diet provides everything your body needs to energize and renew itself. A rapid shift in diet will take some time for your body to adapt to. Dieting without supervision can compound already existing problems, lead to nutritional deficiencies and create additional difficulties simply through the effect of rapid change. Change without preparation involves a shift in psychological patterns, one of the cornerstones of stress. If you are concerned about nutritional deficiencies, consult your physician. Don't self-diagnose or self-treat.

Cigarettes, marijuana, alcohol, and sugar are all examples of immunological suppressants—they can lower your immune system responses. However, the problem really is one of overdoing, especially when there are indications that you should be taking care of yourself. Your body adapts very well to a moderate, constant intake of substances which, if taken in excess or in isolation can depress your immune system resources. While stopping smoking will definitely make you a lot healthier in general and protect you somewhat from lung cancer and cardiac problems, you probably won't see a direct and clear effect on herpes and certainly not for some time. Excess, chronic, and sudden insult to the system is really what we are worried about here. In the simplest terms, don't hurt yourself. Don't burn yourself out too often, especially when you have prodromal signs! Having a good time is one thing—overdoing is another. Incidentally, oversleeping is just as bad as undersleeping. Your body balance gets out of tune.

Keep yourself in reasonable shape. It's irrelevant how, at least as far as herpes is concerned. Do what's good for you to keep your mood, energy and physical well-being in as good condition as possible.

Eating well, sleeping well, exercising well, and acting for your own benefit all interact very strongly with how you think. Here's a good example from someone I know who is in excellent physical shape, a marathon runner who asserted that he could count on an outbreak of herpes a day after a race whether a ten mile race or a twenty-six mile race. His head was set on the idea that really draining his body resources would result in a recurrence. I asked him if he got the same results from his practice races as from his formal ones (not to mention his hundred-odd mile-a-week training regimen). The question was sufficient to interrupt the pattern. When he saw the races as really draining his body's resources and as something detrimental to him, he had an outbreak. He did not think about his training in this way. His mind-set, which included a high load of self-induced anxiety about herpes, was playing a role here. When he realized this, he was able to break the pattern.

Behave well in the sense of knowing what's good for you and what's bad for you and recognize the distinction between self-destruction and what you can take in stride.

Prodromal and Trigger Factors

Gaining control over herpes means two things—first, being able to anticipate events and cope with them; and second, playing a direct role in symptom reduction. There are no guaranteed prescriptions to abort outbreaks, but there are many things that can be done to help reduce the internal and external factors that influence them.

The first step in gaining control is to know your own body. Your body's hormonal, immunological and neural machinery work very much as a dynamic interrelated unit to produce the physical feelings you have as well as your emotional tone, thinking processes, and behavioral patterns. Knowing how your body and mind respond and deal with viral invasion, with life's changes, with happy and sad circumstances is the best source of information for coping with your life in general and herpes in particular. Learn to discriminate among different feelings.

Once you are sensitive to your own body and emotions, your awareness of changes becomes automatic, and you won't need to obsessively observe every sensation. Instead, you will become tuned in to changes related to herpes. You won't even have to think about it, you'll just "know." Later, you'll be able to use that information to shift your personal focus away from herpes. But let's start with that set of initial signs that provide the information you need to begin to gain control over herpes.

The following is a sample of the range of sensations people report. As mentioned in an earlier chapter, you may experience one or several. The aim is to be able to identify the signs associated with herpes outbreaks as far ahead of time as possible.

The symptoms are:
- an itch close to an outbreak area
- a tingling sensation
- a pinprick feeling
- a sensitivity or a feeling that something is about to happen

These usually signal an outbreak itself and occur close to the appearance of the rash. Others include:

○ a pulsing or dull ache in the general area or down one leg or side of the groin

○ a kind of muscular tension or ache such as you might get from exercise

○ hotness or feverishness in the groin area

○ tenderness

○ actual pain, which you may not be able to locate specifically, hidden somewhere in legs, groin, or pelvic area

○ burning or pain on urination or defecation.

The latter set of sensations are sometimes followed by active outbreaks, and sometimes continue for several days or longer before either an outbreak occurs, or the sensations diminish and disappear without an outbreak occurring. These are particularly useful in that they indicate that there is some stress in or on the body, whose source can usually be located and often removed.

Trigger factors are usually identifiable on an individual basis as physical, emotional, or social stresses. Since sunlight is a direct trigger factor for herpes I, a sunscreen is an extremely useful preventive measure. Other physical traumas that hurt or abrade the skin can trigger some genital outbreaks. Massage oil will protect external tissue from the effects of rough handling (don't use it internally), and K-Y jelly will protect internal tissues from abrasion during intercourse. Simple care is the watchword here. Intercourse without adequate lubrication is deliberate intent to destroy tissue.

Dry skin tends to cause a sensitivity that can hasten an impending outbreak of external sores. This can be a problem, expecially in winter in city apartments, where the dry heat helps to maintain a potential irritation. Be gentle with your skin if this is the case. Make sure there is sufficient lubrication during sex and don't use abrasive soaps or overly hot water. A humidifier will help. Eliminating the potential of physical trauma alone is a great preventative for outbreaks for many people and is in keeping with the essence of sexuality—care and concern for what you are doing. And in terms of healing outbreaks, since irritation and aggravation of the area will retard healing time, a little care will eliminate the problem. In hot, humid summer months, wear loose cotton underwear and use unscented talcum powder to help stay dry and cool.

Menstruation can become established as a trigger factor for some women. While viral activation has been linked to hormonal levels or changes, the fact that outbreaks are not coincident with menstruation for most women and that women with a history of outbreaks during menstruation do not always do so, suggests that the link is not direct and can be broken. Again, the goal is to separate herpes from other factors in your life.

Lowered resistance can serve as an invitation for a recurrence. Herpes often breaks out during periods of reduced physical and emotional resources. Regarding this, there are two important things to remember. The first is to keep yourself in good shape. The second is more complicated. If herpes is presently your Achilles heel, it doesn't have to remain so. Beware of the vicious cycle that turns into a destructive habit. While outbreaks are more likely to show up when your body resources are depleted by another infection such as a cold, it's possible to keep the two separate. Herpes can become a serious problem in severely immune-suppressed patients, but that is a rather exceptional circumstance and doesn't apply to the average person.

Your goal is to break the cycle. Herpes doesn't inevitably have to break out when you are a little run down, it is just more likely to.

Stress
As in everything else related to herpes, stress is an individual affair and different for each person. However, there

are several common rules to help identify and remove stressful situations. Let's draw up the relationships between herpes and stress. Working backwards,

o   An event occurs in neural tissue to activate herpes towards an outbreak.

o   Physiological change often plays a role in this "event."

o   The physiological change often occurs as a result of a threat to body or mind. In other words, the body/mind system unconsciously and automatically mobilizes forces to respond to a potentially dangerous situation.

This mobilization of forces occurs along three major lines. One, activation of parts of the nervous system to speed up heart rate, send blood to muscles, and create energy for action—the "fight or flight response." Two, release of hormones to reinforce this nervous system effect, such as adrenaline, or epinephrine. And three, activation of immunological mechanisms.

Neural and hormonal responses occur all the time in short bursts and are essential to you in dealing with day-to-day challenges. The system operates beautifully. When a challenge has passed or has been taken care of, an opposite set of responses comes into play to restore equilibrium— slow things down; conserve energy stores; and rebuild and renew tissue. Your body knows full well what it is doing.

Stress in itself is fine and necessary to life. It promotes growth, renewal and adaptation, both physical and behavioral. We are continually adapting to changing circumstances in our bodies and lives in general. That's the nature of life processes.

The inherent problem, however, is that we can stretch our adaptational capacities just so far before detrimental effects occur. For example, cardiac and blood pressure problems are manifested by physical symptoms but are often related to long periods of continued stress as well as behavior that aggravates the condition. This includes eating particular foods, smoking cigarettes, and sustained tension. The continued stress steps up the neural and hormonal systems a notch or two. A breakdown of adaptational mechanisms occurs as well as a decrease in all body processes that deal with foreign agents or internal changes. This has two effects related to herpes. First, continued neural activation can easily become channeled into herpes activation. Second, sweepup and healing by the immune system will be greatly diminished, resulting in more outbreaks of longer duration.

We cannot remove all stresses from life, but we can do a great deal to alleviate chronic stress and to reduce the channeling of everyday stresses into herpes. But it takes a little looking into. There's a chart included in this chapter to help you identify areas that may be stressful to you, ways in which you may be directly or indirectly hurting yourself through stress, perhaps without even knowing it.

Points to Remember
○ The effects of stressful situations can become channeled into herpes.
○ Since herpes can become a path of least resistance for the body effects of these stresses, a pattern can become established.
○ Chronically stressful situations are dangerous to your health via breakdown of normal recovery processes and depressions of immune defense capabilities.

So where do these stresses come from? How can they be identified? What can you do about them? The effects just outlined are a result of your body and mind working together to perceive a situation or event as potentially threatening or dangerous. If you are able to consciously identify things that can have this effect on you, then you can do something about them. For example, an upcoming job interview is anxiety producing, but good preparation can reduce much of the potentially deleterious effects, whereas leaving everything to the last minute and continually worrying will extend and intensify them.

The insidious thing about stress in relation to herpes is that often the stress response will occur way beneath our awareness and show up as physical symptoms. But we can get a handle on much of this.

Perceptions of Herpes

As we've seen, herpes often has the capacity to elicit feelings such as fear of rejection, anger, and other negative emotions. These in turn can cause a stress response via worry and anxiety, which is often unrecognized. A rather vicious cycle gets established; a herpes outbreak leads to more hidden worry which, in turn, contributes to an outbreak, and so on.

Remember again, herpes is only a small part of your life. You have your life to live by channeling your energies towards more productive pursuits than helping to make viruses! Break that cycle by breaking the link between herpes and negative emotions.

Interpersonal Issues

For many people, the emotional responses and frustrations that can occur with herpes tend to isolate them from others and hence feed into the problem. When you are able to talk about herpes with others who can empathize, you'll break that feeling of isolation. You'll also find that your fear of rejection has significantly diminished.

The quickest and best, although not always the easiest, way to dispense with the rest of the stressful effects of fear of rejection is to have successful interpersonal things happen. The depressive side of fear of rejection, seen in lowered self-esteem and self-confidence, responds best to first very small and gradually larger rewarding personal achievements. Success will breed success, and the important thing is that you have made the successes happen. You are no longer at the mercy of circumstances. Set your goals small and then build on them.

You have broken the back of this problem when you wrest control of events away from herpes and into your own hands. The final step occurs when you apply this approach to interpersonal relationships and work through the "how to tell" problem. Once you take the responsibility and consequences of your actions into your own hands and carry out your plan of action, herpes will not control you. Failures and setbacks are bound to occur, so keep a support system of friends around you for encouragement. People do master the effects of isolation and interpersonal fears. In so doing, you can substantially reduce the stress which can have a very profound effect on symptoms, and your perception of them.

We spoke earlier of another potent source of emotional stress, which concerns conflicting sets of emotions or motivations about relationships—a tendency to choose interpersonal situations that cannot work out. This might simply be a way to keep people at a distance. It is almost the same as withdrawing and partly stems from the same source. Herpes or not, there is a fear of not being up to par or at your best. Being unsure is not something to be ashamed of, but something to be dealt with because herpes can feed in to a person's feeling less desirable. If not properly attended to, this kind of ambivalence and other already existing insecurities can become exacerbated. And the increases of stress can contribute to the physiological changes involved in an outbreak.

However, when conflicts are resolved, the life disrupting problems of herpes are very much curtailed and often, chronic outbreaks are reduced to occasional brief recurrences.

Personal Issues

A more difficult problem for some women to resolve comes from part of our cultural training: Sex and sexual parts are seen in some way as taboo, not to be loved and cared for as part of one's self and one's being. Herpes can add to the associated feelings of lack of worth to create doubt as well as guilt or shame. Certainly anger will occur here. Again, this can be directed in a constructive way to motivate getting on top of herpes, not to mention those culturally ingrained feelings. Separating these feelings from herpes itself is an important aid to all aspects of adjustment.

Men with herpes more often worry about performance. Will it break out before a romantic date? Who will accept a guy who is out of action so often? Again, the doubts and worries can feed on basic questions about self-image which are in turn fed by the culture. When these questions are examined in a rational light—so sometimes you are not in control—this type of stress is removed and adjustment is speeded up.

Emotional responses to herpes are tied to many sources, so stresses, as they relate to herpes, are found in many areas of life.

Life Changes and Planning

Changes in one's life can also cause stress. Some changes are unpredictable while others can be controlled to some extent. Relationship breakups can be very stressful, as can changing jobs or moving. Recognize that all changes require a period of adjustment and, if you can, make one major change at a time and plan as best you can. Then you won't be swept away in an ocean of unpredictable events. Having a sense of control and being able to anticipate and prepare can very much reduce the stresses of change in your life.

The "too busy" syndrome falls under this category.

Some people thrive on a slight overload, while others do not respond as well to having too much to do. Feeling overwhelmed is an indicator to take stock and adjust things accordingly. It is not always easy to organize time more efficiently or to plan further down the road. But if you have no time for enjoyment and reward beyond another apparent achievement, then you are hurting yourself and most likely working on the side of herpes. The "too busy" syndrome can be very well hidden, so take a careful look at your schedule.

How to Reduce Stress

Direct means of reducing immediate stress can be found in various relaxation techniques. I've included some references to different types of methods in the resource section. The key to all of them is giving yourself some time out from mental concerns and physical drain and spending some good time on yourself.

One standard technique is deep muscle relaxation, which has been used successfully in many areas of life and of medicine. It can easily be adapted to help rechannel concerns away from herpes and therefore play a role in symptom reduction. I will give you the outline and you can adjust it according to your needs and personality.

Identifying prodromal signs ahead of time is the first step to starting antioutbreak action. Recognize those signs and use them as a stimulus to begin a relaxation regimen.

> Lie down comfortably. Clench one fist and tense your forearm. Now relax the muscles and feel the relaxation. Don't clench too tightly, just enough to feel the difference when you slowly relax the muscles. Feel the heaviness and warmth set in. Do this with your upper arm, nice and slowly. Then repeat with the other hand and arm.
> Now the legs, one at a time, and then move through the rest of the body—back, abdomen, shoulders, neck and face—tensing and relaxing.

Build on this over a few days until you can relax at will. There are all sorts of ways to learn to relax at will and make peace with your mind. Some people like meditation; there are various forms of meditation to try. Others like to imagine themselves in a beautiful place, while some may have a favorite piece of music to listen to, a picture to visualize, or poem to read. The secret is to have a fixed and constant therapy that will help you to quiet your mind and body. Find the one that works for you and keep at it until you can slip into it at will. Some people generate an image of being in a favorite place. One man I know had the curious (but for him successful) image of fusing three colors together in his mind. When they were all merged together perfectly, he knew he had his body and mind where he wanted them to be. Try creating your own imagery to eliminate herpes sensations.

Let the feelings of relaxation take over your mind and body. Don't try too actively—allow it to happen. You started with herpes prodrome signs, relaxed until the relaxation sensations took over your consciousness, and, if you continue now, you'll be able to eliminate the prodromal sensations from your consciousness. It's possible. In other words, make your perceptions of them disappear. Reinforce this by telling yourself what you are going to do before you start each time. If your pain is more severe than the usual dull ache, this will be more difficult (see the resource section). For most prodromes, however, it is possible to reduce the effects of stress in an outbreak.

Start as early as possible during a prodrome. When you are able to eliminate herpes sensations from your mind, you will have come a long way in breaking any effect of the vicious cycle between herpes and emotions.

You are building a set of new habits, creating a positive cycle that reduces herpes sensations through relaxation. This switches your attention away from herpes and to something else. It can become automatic after a while. Some people have gone so far as to eliminate herpes sensations from one part of the body and pass them on in the form of discomfort to another part of the body. A woman I've counseled becomes more active in her work when she feels a prodrome. Since she's ordinarily a procrastinator, this usually reduces her stress. She even went so far as to consider using herpes as a work inducer but decided that might be more self-destructive than useful.

Some of this may sound strange, but it isn't in light of the fact that emotions can feed into herpes and herpes in turn affect emotions. Unless it is checked, that symbiotic relationship will hinder both the physical and emotional adjustments to herpes.

There is no guarantee that you will automatically be able to stop all outbreaks, but *there is a guarantee that you can go a long way toward reducing tension and worries and creating a sense of well-being and control, which will speed up the natural adaptation process.* That in itself is a big feat. There's every reason to believe that you can play a direct role in manipulating your body processes so that you can reduce the impact of those factors that trigger recurrences.

Points to Remember

O Your goal is to eliminate or reduce any factors that may play a role in reactivations so that you can limit outbreak frequency and duration as quickly as possible. Herpes will then take its proper role in your life because it won't be on your mind so much.

O Physical traumas can be avoided by lubrication and reduction of tissue damage.

O Emotional trauma can be eased by gaining control over interpersonal fears and anxieties, time organization and planning.

Unless there are major physical complications, dealing with these areas should have a large effect in removing hindrances to adjustment, bringing you further towards the point where herpes is nothing more than a minor and occasional annoyance.

If you are having more than your share of coping difficulties and not making headway, don't hesitate to seek counseling. No one should remain in a state of helplessness for long periods of time without progress. Professional services should be considered if you find yourself stuck and unable to manage.

Stress Inventory

Use the following chart to help identify areas in general that may be generating more stress than is good for you, but in particular those that might have any bearing on herpes recurrences. Because of the capacity of herpes to take on emotional overtones, stresses often get channeled in the direction of symptoms.

Sometimes it is not easy to recognize things that are stressing the system above and beyond the normal challenges of everyday life until they are pointed out, and even then we don't always pay attention. Also, stress reacts on different people in different ways. It is really your gut sense of things that is more important than the outside events themselves.

The chart should help you to clue in to areas that could use a little straightening out if they are contributing to herpes symptoms.

Many people who have adjusted to herpes over time find that herpes outbreaks, or better, prodromes, have become their stress indicator, and quite a sensitive one. That is, for them, herpes symptoms let them know that something is awry.

	Job/School	Family
Have there been changes in these areas of your life in the past year?		
Are these challenging to you or a drain on your resources?		
How well have you adjusted to them?		
How well have you coped in the past with similar changes?		
Are there more than normal tensions in these areas at the present?		
Are they resolvable?		
How do you cope with them?		
How much control do you have over them as they affect you?		
Does your strategy for each solve the problem? Put it off? Maintain it?		
How well are you realizing your hopes for the future in these areas?		
Are your expectations realistic and achievable, in the shortrun? the long run?		
Are your throughts about these positive on the whole, or negative?		
Are you on track with your plans?		

Inventory of areas that can provide stresses that feed into herpes symptoms.

Interpersonal relations	Financial	Living arrangements

Here are some other questions to ask yourself:

o Do you take sufficient time for yourself and/or your recreational or vocational interests?

o Does your daily or weekly routine handle nutrition, work, relaxation and social necessities to your liking?

o Do you recognize when you are tense?

o What are your characteristic ways of dealing with frustration or disappointment? Do you respond with assertiveness? Problem-solving capabilities? Procrastination? Do you wait and see what happens? build up anger and resentment? worry quietly? avoid? feel guilty that you did something wrong?

You'll notice that none of the questions mention herpes. There's really only one blanket question for that. How far are you in resolving your relationship with herpes so that coexisting with it is as tension-free as possible?

10
Questions and Answers

The following is a summary of questions and answers about herpes to serve as a guide to all the important areas and concerns. The issues are discussed in the order in which they are usually raised.

Information is your key to controlling herpes. Keep in mind that the facts about herpes require some digestion. Terse answers to nagging questions can leave you feeling unfulfilled though the facts have been provided, an especially true situation with herpes—it can be such an emotionally laden issue since it often touches so directly on sexuality. In my experience, it takes many runs through the facts before they can be taken at face value and used effectively in prevention. But truly understanding the facts will help you live fully and without worry after contracting herpes.

How do I know if I have herpes?

There are so many infections and other problems that can occur in the mouth or genitals that it is bad practice to self-diagnose. See a physician as soon as you notice unusual symptoms. A trained physician can usually distinguish herpes from other problems quite easily when a rash is present. If no rash is present, he or she cannot. A blood test does not identify a rash as herpes. Instead it will show whether or not you have been exposed to herpes at any time in the past by identifying those antibodies your body has produced against it. A more definitive diagnosis can be made by means of a viral culture test. The infected area is swabbed or scraped. This specimen is then placed in a culture medium to see if the virus can be grown. If so, it provides a positive diagnosis.

This is very important because many people think they have herpes when they may have some other problem. On the other hand, many people are running around with undiagnosed herpes. The symptoms will go away in time, but that is not the end of the story.

What causes herpes?

The disease referred to as herpes is caused by a virus. There are actually a group of herpes viruses that are responsible for several different diseases: chicken pox in childhood and shingles in adults (varicella-zoster virus, VZ), infectious mononucleosis (Epstein-Barr virus, EBV), cytomegalic inclusion disease (cytomegalovirus, CMV), and the recurrent rashes of facial and genital herpes (herpes simplex viruses I and II, HSV I and HSV II). These last two types, HSV I and HSV II are what we are concerned with here.

What is the difference between HSV I and HSV II?

While HSV I and HSV II can be separately identified, this has little or no meaning in terms of symptoms. The designation HSV I is used to refer to infections above the waist and HSV II to those below the waist.

Can I get HSV I on the genitals or HSV II on the face?
Yes. The virus that produces a fever blister can also cause genital sores if that is where it enters the body. Similarly, HSV II can cause an infection on the face from the genitals. So far as can be ascertained, it doesn't matter which virus a person becomes infected with, the symptoms will be the same. It is the location where the infection first occurred that is significant, not whether it is HSV I or II.

How is herpes contracted?
Herpes is contracted *only* through direct physical contact with an active infection in another person. An active infection means sores on the skin or mucous membranes of the body containing herpes viruses. Virus contained in these sores can gain access to another person's body through mucous membranes or abrasions in the skin. Therefore, sexual intercourse with someone who has genital sores will most likely result in transmission to the genitals of the other person. Similarly, kissing a person who has a herpes cold sore will most probably cause an infection on the face or in the mouth of the other person.

If I have a history of cold sores will I get genital herpes?
The herpes infections you will get will be localized to the area initially infected. To get a genital infection from facial sores, you would have to physically put the virus there. In other words, it will not run through your body to suddenly show up on the genitals.

Will having cold sores protect me from getting another kind of herpes infection?
While there is some evidence that a history of herpes might afford some protection from other herpes inoculations (contact with the virus), it is quite clear that people can get more than one infection in different locations. It is possible to have HSV I on the lips and HSV II on the genitals and even another HSV I or II infection somewhere else. It is uncommon, but possible. Getting herpes from one person does not leave you immune to infections from others.

Can I get herpes from oral sex?

Herpes can be transmitted from an active lip infection to the genitals of another person during oral sex. Similarly oral sex with a person who has genital sores present will result in facial or mouth herpes in the other person. Again, herpes is transmitted by direct physical contact. The part of the body that comes in contact with any herpes infection is the part that will become infected.

Can I get herpes in any other way than by sex?

Since direct physical contact is the means of transmission, you can get herpes by touching active sores in another person. This is how some people get herpes on the finger and others in contact sports such as wrestling get herpes on other body areas. But by far the most common means is through kissing and sexual intercourse. You cannot get herpes just being around someone who is broken out in a rash. You must touch the sores directly.

Can I get herpes from toilet seats or water glasses?

It is almost impossible. The herpes virus dies as soon as it leaves the body tissue. While it is a good idea to separate towels, toothbrushes, food and drinking utensils when someone in the family has herpes sores, the chance of infection by these routes is essentially zero. Precautions, however, will relieve anxiety.

Are some people immune to herpes infections?

Some people seem better able than others to withstand herpes inoculations. Similarly, infections in different people will have different degrees of severity.

What factors play a role in the transmission of herpes from one person to another?

The things of importance are:

○ How much virus a person was exposed to
○ That person's constitution—how he or she characteristically is built to respond to a herpes virus invasion.
○ The state of resistance. Run-down people are more likely to succumb to infection than are healthy people

with a full quota of resources. It's like getting colds.

How can I protect myself from getting herpes?

o Use a condom with a new sex partner if you suspect a chance of exposure to any sexually transmissible infection. (However, condoms can protect only the areas covered. If there are sores on the genitals outside the area covered by the condom, transmittal is possible.

o Know your partner. Will he or she willingly or carelessly hurt you?

o Look. If your partner has a cold sore, don't kiss or allow oral sex. Take time to get to know and enjoy your partner's body before intercourse. The virus does not penetrate the skin but requires an abrasion or mucous membranes to inoculate the body. If you come across something that should not be there, ask!

o Ask anyway.

If I am having an outbreak of genital herpes, will using a condom protect my partner?

Using a condom when there are active sores present is not a good idea. The sores will most likely be aggravated, the infection spread, and healing retarded. Best to avoid intercourse until the sores are gone.

What happens when herpes is contracted?

We have to distinguish between a primary (first time) infection and recurrent attacks. In a primary exposure to herpes, the symptoms may be very slight or quite severe depending on a variety of factors including amount of virus, state of health, and constitution.

Typically, symptoms will show between two and twenty days after contact. A rash will develop where contact occurred. If this was in the genital region, it will show as red patches with blister-like white sores on or around the genital area. You may or may not also experience a swelling and tenderness in the groin; pain or burning on urination; a vaginal discharge; fever and general discomfort.

This initial illness will last between two and three weeks in most cases. Then the sores will heal, new skin will grow over the area, and there will be no scarring or residual effects.

Can I get herpes internally?

Yes. You can get herpes in the mouth or throat, vagina or cervix, and anus. These all have mucous membranes that allow passage of the virus into the body. If this occurs, the other general symptoms also will most likely occur.

What are recurrences?

Recurrences refer to times when the herpes rash reappears, apparently from nowhere, at the site where the initial infection occurred. This doesn't happen for everyone. Many people have only one bout with herpes and no future rashes. With others, the rash periodically reappears, perhaps three to five times a year (less for many). Recurrences, on the whole, are much less severe than primary infections and usually last between four and ten days.

Why is herpes recurrent?

Recurrences happen with herpes because it is a virus that can go into a dormant or latent phase in the body. Latent means hidden, and dormant you can take to mean something like sleeping or inactive. Wart viruses can do this. After a wart has been replaced by new skin, the virus still resides in the body.

How does herpes become dormant?

Herpes is a clever virus that escapes body defenses by entering the nearest nerve cells where it is safe from annihilation by the immune system. When body defenses begin to kill off cells invaded by the virus and tissue is regenerated to heal the sores, some viruses escape, then migrate away from the skin surface to become sleeping partners in the cells' nuclei. There is no rash and no virus at the surface and for all intents and purposes no other indication that it is present at all. In this state it cannot be transmitted.

How do recurrences happen?

Under particular conditions, the virus will begin to retrace its migration path back toward the skin surface to infect surface cells and cause another rash.

What factors are important in recurrences?

There are four major factors:

o   Physical trauma (in the form of sunlight) can facilitate facial sores.

o   Abrasions of the skin or mucous membranes are factors in all types of sores.

o   Sudden physiological changes in body balance (all types of sores).

o   Emotional stress (all types).

We don't understand specifically how or why the virus decides to come out of its latent state or how physical or emotional trauma can help trigger reactivations. But these four are the most common contributors to reactivations. If they are present, they will also tend to prolong the healing process once a recurrence has begun.

Why do some people have recurrences more often than others or for longer periods of time?

There are many individual factors operating. They include physical constitution, life-style, and ways of coping with the world in general. In severe cases, with chronic outbreaks, other factors, such as a nutritional or immunological deficienty or poor response to chronic stress may be factors and should be attended to professionally.

Are there any other medical complications associated with herpes?

Yes, but before outlining them, I want to impress upon you that they can all be dealt with easily with a little bit of care. So get the facts, use them and then drop most of the worry.

HERPES KERATITIS. Infections of the eyes can be contracted directly as in other herpes infections and by self-transfer of the virus through picking it up on the finger and rubbing the eye. This is a very rare occurrence with recurrent herpes and essentially unheard of from genital herpes, because of the location of the sores. It is more common from primary facial herpes.

CANCER. Herpes virus has been linked statistically with cancer of the cervix. The risk for cervical cancer is five to eight times greater when a woman has genital herpes. However, greater statistical risk is associated with factors such as beginning sexual intercourse at an early age, having many sex partners, or having uncircumcised partners. The potential for cervical cancer can be dealt with by having Pap smears taken once every six months. If a precancerous abnormality shows up, the treatment is fairly simple and highly effective.

In rare cases, the herpes virus causes encephalitis in adults, occurring through a process called neurogenic spread. It is linked only to facial and oral herpes. Herpes does not cause sterility, pelvic inflammatory disease or neural dysfunctions. While some people will experience various degrees of discomfort during recurrences, there are no residual physical problems or permanent difficulties.

What about pregnancy?

The only issue to consider is whether or not herpes lesions are present in a woman's genitals during delivery because the baby could pick up the virus while passing through the birth canal. In rare cases, the newborn can develop encephalitis by picking up the herpes virus. Newborns have little defense against infection and spread of the virus can occur rapidly so that brain tissue becomes infected. Your obstetrician can monitor you throughout the pregnancy. If no virus is present at term, there is no problem and delivery will be normal. If there is, a Caesarean section will be recommended, and the baby will be protected. The virus does not travel up the birth canal to cross the placenta. A good relationship with your gynecologist or obstetrician serves the purpose of removing all risks to your baby so far as herpes is concerned. After the baby is born, be careful of transmission. Don't let the baby come in contact with herpes sores. And that's all—otherwise, everything is as normal.

Does herpes cause impotency or lack of desire?

Not directly. But it can very much do so via natural emotional responses. The big issue here is based on a fear of rejection that manifests itself in many ways. Herpes sufferers sometimes experience fears of not being acceptable, virile, attractive, desirable, and so on. The best way to think about herpes is in a problem-solving manner. Herpes is another problem to be dealt with in as direct and creative a way as possible. Remember these are feelings, not physical realities, regardless of what other less-informed people may think or what impressions the media may give.

Herpes is not you. You just have a rash that occasionally gets in the way. When you can handle the contagion problem, the emotional concerns will diminish. People with herpes can make love, do make love, and make and break relationships for the same reasons as anyone else. Let's throw any stigmas associated with herpes out the window. It's the best way to break the link between herpes virus and your emotions.

How do I know when I am contagious?

In most cases there are many signs, *prodromal* signs, that an outbreak may be imminent. Learn to identify what is going on in your body with regard to outbreaks. When there is potential for spread, the golden rule is: Don't have any part of anyone's body touch the infected area. You can do anything you like so long as this is observed! When genital sores are present, abstinence from sexual intercourse is the most appropriate preventive measure. Using condoms at this time will most likely simply prolong healing because of the irritation of sores, and of course condoms can only protect the areas covered. There are many other ways to share sexual intimacies beyond intercourse.

When there is a rash, assume you are contagious. Other signs vary with each individual and may include:

- itching sensations
- aches in the groin or surrounding muscles
- tenderness or hotness in the groin area
- a neuralgia in the pelvis or leg, the feeling of a nerve being stimulated

If you can identify your particular signs, then you have a handle on what is going on in your body. You can use these signs first to identify when precautions might need to be observed, and secondly, as indications that something stressful is happening to your body that you may be able to do something about (see later question on stress).

How can I prevent against potential physical complications?

Precautions against potential physical complications are easy to apply:

- After cleaning and drying sores, wash your hands and keep them away from the lesions.
- Exercise good hygiene.
- Women who suffer from herpes should have a good and open relationship with their gynecologist and or obstetrician and have Pap tests done every six months.

After you handle the physical facts, know that there is often a strong interaction between a person's having herpes and their emotional relationship to the world. Recognize how your feelings may be affected by having contracted herpes.

In what ways can herpes affect people emotionally?

If it were only the physical dimensions of genital herpes that we had to deal with there would not be so much concern. It is not a life-threatening affair.

In recurrences, symptoms, for the most part, are not seriously debilitating except in special cases. However, the anxieties about contagion initially can curtail freedom in forming or maintaining relationships.

It is crucially important to recognize that this can happen. Because of the feeling that an unpredictable block may arise to get in the way of intimacy, some people get very frightened. In fact, very few people are immune to at least some of the emotional concerns about relationships. Unfortunately, this can snowball to become worse than the virus itself. It's important to recognize if and when this is happening. Herpes is contagious for short periods once in a while. If symptoms are more severe than this after the body has had time to adapt, then there is something else wrong and professional help should be sought. But, the initial adjustment period for people can be quite difficult if little information is available, and particularly if there is no one to discuss concerns with.

We are dealing with both a physical adaptation process over time and an adjustment in life-style to accommodate the precautions necessary to prevent spread or complications.

Can I be a carrier of herpes without knowing it?

Since most of the United States population shows antibodies to either HSV I or II, then a very large number of people are carriers of the latent virus. But the latent virus cannot be transmitted to someone else.

Herpes can cause mild infections that may go unnoticed. Identifiable recurrences may or may not occur from such infections. There is some evidence of asymptomatic viral shedding in a very small minority of women, and small amounts of the virus have been picked up by culture tests when these women did not display or report rashes. Also, the virus has been picked up in the saliva of both men and women.

It is not possible to determine whether or not sufficient virus was present in these cases to cause an infection in another person, and there have been no documented cases of infections occurring from this type of viral shedding. If it occurs at all, its incidence is very low. Herpes transmission is undoubtedly due primarily to transmission by people who are poorly informed and are therefore unaware of or are ignoring symptoms that do exist. They have herpes that has never been diagnosed.

Informed partners very rarely infect one another. This couldn't be the case if asymptomatic viral shedding was significant in transmission. With mutual cooperation, the risk of transmitting herpes to a partner is negligible.

Unfortunately, this issue can, for some people, become overly significant emotionally, which creates feelings of contamination or of being in a constant state of contagion. It is important to recognize that these are only feelings and not realities. Do not let them interfere with closeness and intimacy.

Why is there no cure for herpes?

The tremendous technical problem is to find a substance that can chase the virus into its nerve cell retreat. It is relatively easy to kill the virus when it has surfaced, and many compounds will do that, but eradicating it in its dormant form is another matter. So while there are many treatments for killing the virus at the surface of the skin, none can be guaranteed to prevent recurrences because the dormant source cannot be attacked.

What about all the treatments that are advertised in newspapers and magazines?

These are ways to steal money, not to cure people. Many of them can be dangerous to your general health and despite their claims, none of them ultimately work. Herpes is a ubiquitous disease that can, in certain circumstances, be very open to suggestion and especially hope. Zovirax, a new antiviral, has been recently approved by the FDA. It reduces viral shedding in a herpes outbreak and may shorten its duration by up to a day. But it cannot affect the virus in its latent form and so cannot prevent recurrences. If you are sufficiently primed for success, there is no doubt that almost any new treatment will prevent or abort one or two outbreaks. But the long-range adaptation is most likely retarded either through the new treatment itself or the physiological changes resulting from bombarding your body with many different and potent substances. On top of that, the ensuing disappointments will help neither your herpes, nor your mood and adjustment.

What can I do to control herpes myself?

This is a two-pronged question. First, knowing about contagion and being able to recognize contagion signs means that you can plan and/or work around the problem. This is called adjustment. Secondly, you can do a great deal to prevent recurrences. Removing physical trauma when there is potential for an outbreak is very effective. Reducing physical factors that don't help your body and reducing stress by using more effective coping strategies for events you have to deal with will all significantly reduce the potential for recurrences.

How are outbreaks related to stress?

Herpes can sometimes become the Achilles heel of your body in that any challenges your body has difficulty dealing with can become channeled in the direction of herpes activation. This is a rather unfortunate link that can become established, meaning that any kind of stressful situation in work or school, social or family life, interpersonal life and so on might feed into herpes symptoms. Sometimes anxieties can be well hidden but nonetheless have their effect. Removing these stressors and/or breaking the link between them and herpes symptoms has a very large effect on recurrences.

What can I do about stress in relation to herpes?

First, see if you can identify events, situations, behavior and thoughts that seem related in your own life to imminent herpes activity. There's a chart included earlier for that purpose. Then you have a chance to do something about these things. The goal here is to gain some control of the effects of stressful situations on your life. You cannot remove the challenges you are beset with; however, you can do something about how they affect you. Also, find ways to spend some good time with yourself every day by relaxing or doing something you enjoy or that is rewarding to you in a very personal way. If you don't have time for that, then you are automatically under stress.

The Basic Points to Remember About Herpes

○ Information and understanding are the keys to control of herpes and of its spread.
○ Contagion and the potential for physical complications are quite easy to take care of with a minimum of care and good hygiene.
○ Recognition of the ways in which herpes can interfere with our sexual feelings and feed on fears goes a long way in reducing herpes to its proper perspective and preventing its interference in life and love.

But most of all:

○ People with herpes have emotionally and sexually fulfilling relationships that produce joy and passion and healthy babies.

Have I succeeded in getting my experience with the herpes problem across to you? Then you are either well prepared to avoid the pitfalls that herpes can present, should you contract it, or well on your way to a quick adjustment and control over it should you and herpes already have met.

Further Resources

Should you need it, the following books and audio tapes will provide further help with coping in general. Write to the publisher or supplier for details about each to help choose which will be most useful to you.

Books

Benson, H. The Relaxation Response. New York: William Morrow & Co. Inc., 1975.

Jacobsen, L. You Must Relax. New York: McGraw-Hill Inc., 1962.

Lazarus, R. S. Psychological Stress and the Coping Process. New York: McGraw-Hill Inc., 1966.

Olshan, N. H. Power Over Pain Without Drugs. New York: Rawson, Wade Inc., 1981.

Pelletier, K. H. Mind as Healer, Mind as Slayer. New York: Delta Books, 1977.

Simonton, O. C., Matthews-Simonton, S., and Creighton, J. Getting Well Again. Los Angeles: J. P. Tarcher Inc., 1978.

TAPES

"Progressive Relaxation: Gross Muscles/Fine Muscles," tape #101;

"Self-directed Relaxation/Spacial Relaxation," tape #102;

"Guided Imagery Relaxation/Breathing Relaxation," tape #103;

Conscious Living Foundation, P.O. Box 513, Manhattan, Kansas, 66502.

"Meditation and Behavioral Self-Management," Cat. #T-128B;

"Rational Emotive Self-Help Techniques," Cat. #T-36B;

"Self-Modification of Anxiety: Client Instructions," Cat. #T-44B; BMA Audio Cassettes, 200 Park Avenue So., New York, New York 10003

The Herpes Resource Center

By far the best source of information about all issues related to herpes is The Herpes Resource Center, a program service of the American Social Health Association. The address is Herpes Resource Center, P.O. Box 100, Palo Alto, CA. 94302.

The Herpes Resource Center publishes *The Helper*, a quarterly journal devoted to herpes that provides up-to-date information on research and political activities related to herpes and a forum for concerns of people who have herpes, among other valuable services.

The Center sponsors research, conferences, and workshops, and promotes activities to further speed up the process of finding an ultimate cure for herpes.

On the more personal side, it coordinates a nationwide program for people with herpes, which to date has some fifty-odd local self-help chapters where people can discuss common concerns and help each other with any difficulties encountered in coping with herpes. Check the *Yellow Pages* for your local office.

Overall, the Herpes Resource Center has developed a well-coordinated attack on the herpes problem. You can become a member by writing to the above address. You will receive *The Helper* and access to a national Helpline, a hotline established specifically to answer questions about herpes, and to local and national activities related to herpes.

Index

A
Acetone, 52
Alcohol (drinking), 23, 74
Alcohol (rubbing), 18, 52
American Social Health Association (ASHA), 3
AMP (drug), 52
Analgesics, 17
Antibiotics, 44
Antibodies, 32, 44
See also Immune system
Antiviral agents, 47-49
See also individual agents
Ara-A (antiviral), 48

B
Bacterial infections, 21, 40
Bathing (and rash), 23
BCG (drug), 50
Betadine, 49
Burow's solution, 23

C
Cervical cancer, 41-42
Cigarettes, 23
and body's resistance, 74
Communication between partners, importance of, 37-38
Condoms, 32, 38, 95
Corticosteroids, 49

D
DMSO (drug), 51
Dye-light treatment, 51

E
Emotional problems (and herpes), 55-71
Ether, 52

G
General health, 9, 16, 23, 26, 74-75, 78

H
Herpes
advertised treatments for, 102
burning and, 9, 77
common questions about, 91-104
contagion, 8, 27-38, 93, 94, 99
See also physical contact and transmission
course of infection, 8-11
cure, impossibility of, 1-2, 11, 25, 102
diagnosis, 8, 92
discomfort, 16
discussing with partner, 63-72
examples of, 65-68
embarrassment and, 57
emotions and, 1, 57-62, 100
exposure, degree of, 94
in the eyes, 40-41, 97
See also Herpes keratitis
facial, 6, 7
See also HSV I
fear and, 58-59, 109
fear of rejection, 81
general health and, 9, 16, 23, 26, 74-75, 78
genital, 6, 7, 9
See also HSV II
glands, swollen and, 9
hygiene and, 22-23, 26
ignoring, 2
immune system and, 10, 11, 32, 50, 74-75, 78
and impotence, 99
inflammation, 16
itching, 9, 76
latency and, 11-13, 32, 43
permanent nature of, 12
location of infection, 6
media and, 3, 102
irresponsibility of, 3, 57
medical complications of, 39-44, 97, 100
medical treatment, 39-44, 97, 100
necessity of, 10, 11
research in, 46
myths, 1, 3
oral sex and, 94
pain and, 15-20
treatment, 17-20
personal problems and, 55-62, 83-84
physical contact and, 7, 28, 31
See also contagion and transmission
placebo effect and, 23-25
pregnancy and, 42-44
death of infant in, 43
nursing, 44
prevention, 35-38, 95
primary infection, 11, 95